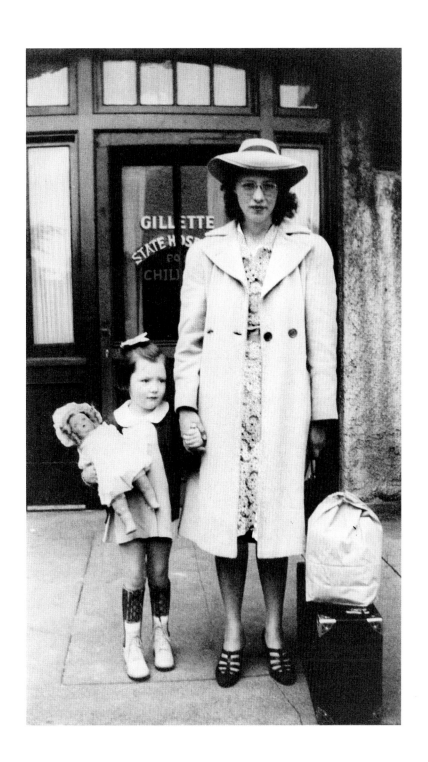

We Hold This Treasure

The Story of Gillette Children's Hospital

Here are stories of hope, stories of people willing to spend the treasure of their self, to the betterment of others.

[signature]

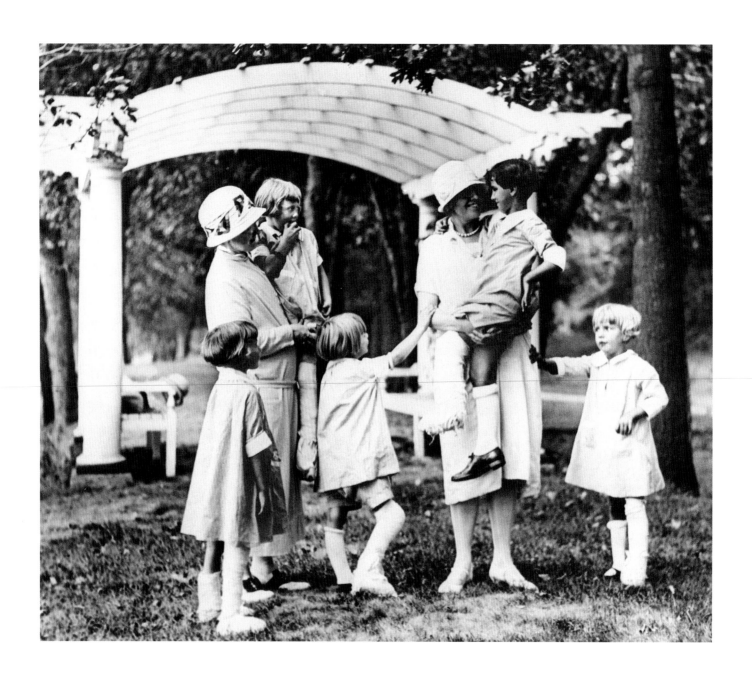

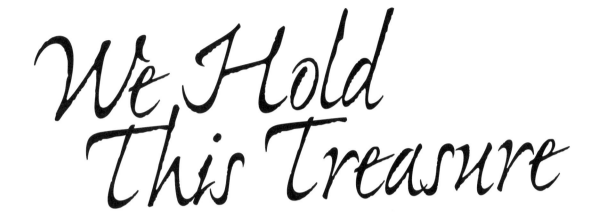

We Hold This Treasure

The Story of Gillette Children's Hospital

STEVEN E. KOOP, M.D.

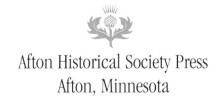

Afton Historical Society Press
Afton, Minnesota

Cover photograph: A nurse reading to children, circa 1920
Half title page: Jean (Schilling) Legried going home with Mom, 1942
Frontispiece: Miss Elizabeth McGregor and Mrs. Katherine Gillette at annual picnic, 1925
Opposite Contents: A nurse charting, circa 1920
Opposite Appendices: Boys with a sheep cart, 1927
Back page: Spine braces with leg extensions, circa 1930
Back cover: Henry Gustafson and a fellow patient, 1927

Designed by Barbara J. Arney

Library of Congress Cataloging-in-Publication Data
Koop, Steven E., 1953–
    We hold this treasure : the story of Gillette Children's Hospital
  / Steven E. Koop. -- 1st ed.
        p.   cm.
    Includes bibliographical references and index.
    ISBN 1-890434-03-5
    1. Gillette Children's Hospital--History.   2. Children--Hospitals-
-Minnesota--St. Paul--History.   I. Title.
    RJ27.3.M6K66   1998   97-26380
    362.1 ' 9892 ' 0009776581--DC21   CIP

Printed in Canada

The Afton Historical Society Press is a non-profit organization that takes great pride and pleasure in publishing fine books on Minnesota subjects.

W. Duncan MacMillan   Patricia Condon Johnston
president   publisher

This book is dedicated to Debbie,
my wife and companion in all that I do,

Brendan, Colin, Allison, and Evan,
our energetic children,

and Stevie,
a light along the journey.

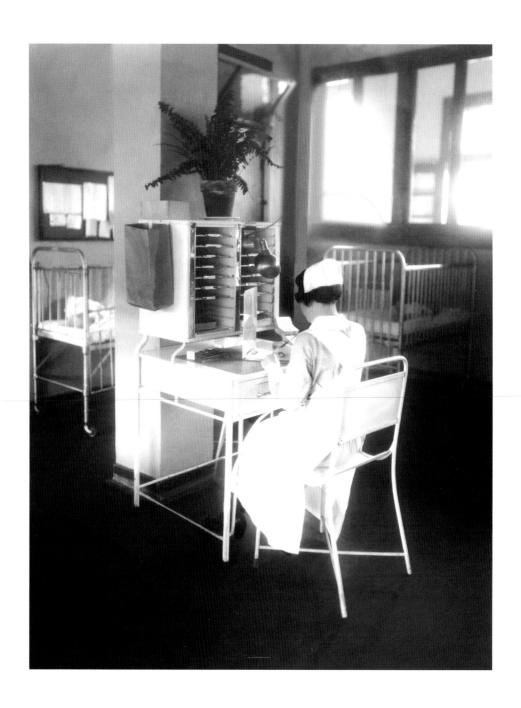

Contents

Preface

We hold this treasure in earthen vessels,
to show that the transcendent power
belongs to God and not to us.

We are afflicted in every way,
but not crushed;
perplexed, but not driven to despair;
persecuted, but not forsaken;
struck down, but not destroyed.

Letter from Paul of Tarsus to the people of Corinth
2 Corinthians 4:7-9

If the title of this book leads you to believe it is about crippled children who are little treasures who deserve our pity, you might be surprised. Instead, you will read the stories of children who were formed differently or changed by injury or illness, and you also will read the stories of those who tried to help them. Many of the children felt struck down and afflicted, and some of them experienced persecution and grew up perplexed. The people who worked with them were not perfect, but the best of them possessed a real treasure: the ability to serve children in need of hope. Perhaps by listening to these stories you will discover the same treasure within yourselves.

In 1982 I spent six months at Gillette Children's Hospital as an orthopaedic resident, or physician-in-training. Residents were expected to complete a research project and Dr. Robert Winter graciously allowed me to study a small group of his patients. While completing this work I discovered that the hospital had preserved all patient records in their original form beginning with the first child treated in

1897. Those records fascinated me, for many of them spanned an entire childhood. Most of my project time was spent examining x-rays, but I was more interested in each child's story. My research was published in an orthopaedic medical journal but my real discovery was the collection of old patient records. I came to view those 50,000 records as a chorus of human experiences.

I returned to Gillette as a staff physician in 1985. I wanted to explore the old records but I was busy with patients. During those years, however, the staff in the medical records department asked me to respond to letters from past patients, many of whom had received care before 1960. I invited those former patients to return to the hospital, and some came to visit. Most of them wanted to know more about their childhood problems and I showed them their records and explained the treatment they had received. The records and the photographs they contained released powerful emotions and memories. Those visits pushed me to organize a review of all of the hospital's patient records.

My first goal was to create a database that would allow the hospital to understand its history and to conduct studies of long-term outcomes of medical care. I started by considering what information should be placed in such a database and settled on four categories. The first category contained basic demographic information, such as names, addresses, and so forth. The second category included diagnoses the children had been given, and the third described surgical procedures performed for each child. The last category was a listing of all images associated with the children, including x-rays, photographs, movies, and newer tests such as magnetic resonance scans. Once the content of the database was settled the real work began.

I knew it was not possible for me to review all the records and still work as a physician. In 1989 I employed Kathy McCarty to help me, and later Christine (Tina) Given and Darla Stewart joined the group. Dana Dahl worked with us during two summer vacations. Beginning with the first patient records of 1897 we read each file and abstracted pertinent information for the demographic, diagnoses, procedures, and images files. We applied current diagnosis codes to each patient, and found ourselves revising some previous diagnoses. The surgical procedures proved to be a challenge as current procedural terminology often did not apply to surgeries done in the first half of this century. We used the basic elements of modern diagnosis and procedure coding schemes, then modified them to fit our needs. It took six years to read the records and abstract and store the information.

During those years Kathy, Tina, and Darla learned to be patient with me. Our office often resembled an anthill. Every open area was filled with stacks of archive boxes, and we found each other through narrow passageways lined with brown cardboard. When I had time I pulled out boxes of old records, read the corresponding abstracts, made changes if needed, and answered questions when there was uncertainty. My secret delight was watching the staff grow in their passion for the project. They may have started out thinking they had an interesting job but they became ardent converts to the importance of what we were doing.

I thought a database would be sterile if we didn't know something more about the lives of the people who had spent part of their childhood at the hospital. In 1993

I drafted a letter inviting past patients or their family members to contact us for an interview about their experiences. The letter was printed in the "Letters to the Editor" section of every newspaper published in Minnesota. I hoped to hear from thirty or forty people, and was astonished by the response to the invitation. To date we have conducted more than a hundred formal oral history interviews of past patients or employees and received extensive correspondence from more than 300 additional past or current patients.

The oral histories and correspondence convinced me that a book needed to be written, and the hospital's centennial in 1997 provided me with a deadline to complete the task. Many hospital histories have been written but they tend to focus on the doctors and don't say much about the patients. This is not surprising, since most hospitals provide care to adults. By the time a historian becomes interested in the work of a hospital the patients have moved away or have died, or the records have been destroyed. Gillette Children's Hospital was different. Documents had been preserved, large numbers of past patients were alive and living in Minnesota, and it was clear they wanted to talk about their experiences.

In order to write a history of the hospital I needed to learn more about its creation and the people who had worked there. I heard many stories as a resident about past events, but I suspected that some might be inaccurate. Although the hospital had retained a large number of documents, we supplemented them by studying the materials held in the historical collections I have listed in the Notes. This part of the work was particularly fascinating and made us all feel like detectives. We followed hints and clues and found things which sent us off in new directions. Even now I know we haven't found everything. Somewhere out there sits a box of photographs or letters

I could have used but didn't find in time. This thought drives me crazy, but history is always a work in progress.

Throughout our research we have protected the confidentiality of past and present patients of the hospital. At any point in the book where a specific patient is identified in writing, quoted, or portrayed in a photograph I have received written permission from that person. There are two exceptions to that rule: One is the hospital's first patient, Royal Gray, whose name and health problem already had been published. The other exception is photographs of groups of children at the hospital. Most of those photos were of social activities or public events there. They were found in various archives, and the source of each photograph is cited. Occasionally the consequences of certain diseases or disorders were portrayed in photographs where the patient's name was not included. In those it is impossible to identify the patient since the images displayed the problem in the most discreet manner possible.

I owe thanks to many people for their support over the last seven years. Kathy McCarty brought structure to the data base and was a whiz with computers. Tina Given created a system to index and store all the documents found in archives. Darla Stewart made our past patients and employees feel comfortable and welcome during their oral history interviews. All of the team members participated in abstracting old records. Kathy and Tina spent a lot of time and energy pursuing odd documents and bits of information that I thought might be important, and along the way they made valuable discoveries. This book would still be a dream without them. If only every researcher or historian could work with such skilled and dedicated researchers as Kathy, Tina, and Darla. Denise Ricos, my secretary, kept my days organized and under control. I would be lost without her. Patrick Hallock made the database talk to us, Angie Denny was our guide through the old medical records, and her sister, Elaine Smith, cheerfully helped us with research in Spokane, Washington. Ken Jandl and Anna Bittner helped us preserve the photographs which bring the people in this book to life. Margaret Perryman, the chief executive officer of Gillette, and her administrative staff were bemused by my insistence that the archive of old records was a treasure, but they were unfailing in their kindness and support. The Andersen Foundation generously supported a portion of the costs of publishing this book.

Special thanks are reserved for three people. Virginia Brainard Kunz edited my manuscript and gently guided my efforts to write simple and clear sentences. My mother would have said that Virginia had the toughest job. Barbara Arney designed the book and made it a pleasure to hold and read. Most importantly, Patricia Condon Johnston of the Afton Historical Society Press believed in me and in this story. Her quiet encouragement meant a lot to me.

This book was written for the people who were patients at the hospital. I thought it was essential to listen to their stories, acknowledge their experiences, and learn from them. The hospital may be one hundred years old, but it is alive and vibrant. If we are to serve the children of the next century well, we must change where necessary while adhering to enduring principles. In the stories of the last 100 years we may find the places to change and the places to stand fast.

Of Passion and Experience

In the harsh winter months of late 1895 a man from St. Paul came to Northfield, Minnesota, to appeal for help for the homeless. He spoke at a church service and described the special need to find homes for children. He illustrated his message by describing a crippled child who had a pleasing personality but was unwanted because of his deformities.

In the audience that evening was Jessie Haskins, a student at Carleton College. The call of the speaker reached directly into Jessie's heart, for she had a large and noticeable curvature of the spine, and could understand the plight of this crippled child. The speaker could not have anticipated the events that were to follow his presentation.[1]

Jessie responded immediately and sought people to help the cause of homeless children. She first turned to the faculty at Carleton. She had every right to expect a sympathetic response. The college began originally as a preparatory school called Carleton Academy, formed by the State Association of Congregational Churches in Minnesota at its annual meeting in 1866. A trustee group for the academy, which opened in September 1867, was formed from members of the Association. The trustees incorporated Carleton as an educational institution that became independent of control by the Association. By the 1870s the academy had grown to include a four-year college, with its first class graduating in 1874.[2]

From its beginning Carleton had a remarkable faculty and a challenging curriculum. Typical academy classes included Greek, Latin, rhetoric, and algebra. College classes continued education in the classics by studying Cicero, Virgil, and Homer, along with languages, history, sociology, philosophy, and the Bible. A strong women's department existed, headed by Margaret Evans who had earned a doctorate in English literature. Logic and elocution were taught for twenty-seven years, from 1879 to 1906, by the Reverend George Huntington. Several faculty members held graduate degrees in divinity, as exemplified by the Reverend A. H. Pearson who taught chemistry for ten years after earning scientific degrees at Amherst and the Massachusetts Institute of Technology. He was then appointed professor of philosophy and drew upon the divinity studies he had completed at Hartford Theological Seminary for his classroom lectures. The Carleton faculty also was involved in the surrounding community. From October 1895 through April 1896, Professor Pearson delivered twelve lectures on the theory and practice of Bible instruction to the Young Men's Christian Association (YMCA) in Minneapolis. His topics included such lectures as "The Motives to Service" and "The Fields of Service."[3] It is likely that Jessie turned to faculty members such as Pearson, Huntington, and Evans for advice.

It is almost certain that Pearson was a friend of Hastings Hart, the secretary of the Minnesota Board of Corrections and Charities created by the legislature in 1883 at the suggestion of Governor Lucius Hubbard. The board was authorized to examine the whole system of public charities as well as jails and prisons. Hart, who held a divinity degree, was widely recognized for his diligence and his nonpartisan administration of the board.[4] A bulletin was published by the board, and annual meetings held around the state attracted large numbers of people to discuss the state's charitable activities. In March 1896 a letter to the editor entitled "An Institution for Deformed and Crippled Children" appeared in the Minnesota Bulletin of Corrections and Charities. Its author was J.A.H. of Northfield, the initials of Jessie Alice Haskins. Its essential message can be found in a single sentence: "Something should be done to provide schools for deformed and crippled children."

Jessie's letter outlined a persuasive argument to support her position. She noted that the state already had institutions for the blind and deaf, and that students from those schools did well compared to the able-bodied. She also noted that great progress had been made in Europe in the treatment of spine and hip disorders, but that only two or three cities in the United States possessed doctors with those skills, and the poor did not have access to them. The result, Jessie wrote, was that "children that could have been easily cured at first grow up uncared for and gradually grow worse and worse until they are incurable." This seemed intolerable: "Surely these children have a right to have proper schools provided for them." Her conclusion was emphatic: "We should have state institutions where these children could have the latest scientific treatment and their education could progress under more favorable circumstances than in the public schools."[5]

What was the source of such passion? How could a college student listening to a plea for compassion at a church service in a small town write such a cogent letter?

Jessie Haskins was born January 27, 1866, in Oswego, New York, the last of the five daughters

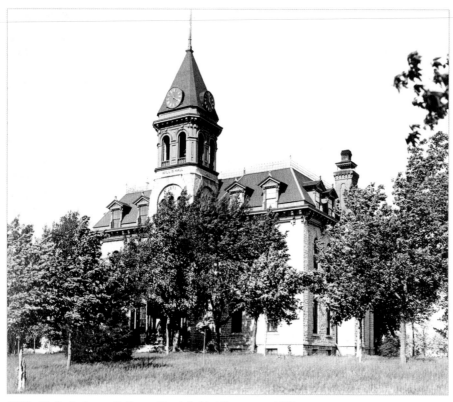

Willis Hall, Carleton College, Northfield, Minnesota, 1900

2

of Hiram and Laurena (Eason) Haskins. Her parents were natives of Oswego County and moved many times during their marriage as Hiram sought employment.

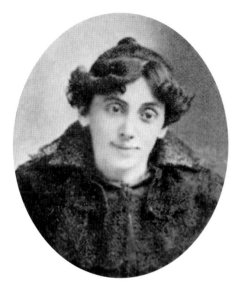

Jessie Alice Haskins, 1899

He sometimes went off alone to work, and he joined the army during the Civil War. Both parents were deeply religious, and Hiram dutifully recorded in his Bible the major events in his family's life. In it Laurena saved some of his letters. Jessie was born six months after her father's death in July 1865.[6] Early in life she developed a deformity of the spine, and despite her mother's attempts, no useful treatment was found. It's possible that Jessie's curvature was the result of tuberculosis, but no one who described her ever reported the sharp rounding of the spine that was typical of Pott's disease, or tuberculosis of the spinal column. She did not have tuberculosis in any major joints and was generally healthy.[7]

Her sister Ella (Haskins) Holly, writing of Jessie many years later,

attributed the spinal curvature to an injury sustained as an infant. She described Jessie as "a very pretty girl with great dark eyes which sparkled and laughed when she was animated, or were veiled in sensitive sadness in her somber moments." Behind the dark, sparkling eyes, Jessie was conscious of her altered appearance, even though other people thought the curve was not particularly noticeable. The curvature, said Ella, "though not very pronounced, caused her much suffering in her childhood, and great mental distress as well, as she grew older and realized that she could not do many of the things which she would have loved." According to Ella, the family reacted protectively: "[Jessie] was so sensitive on the subject that it was never mentioned before her by the family, and we resented with a touch of indignation any mention of it by others to us."[8]

In the early 1870s Jessie's mother moved to St. Paul, bringing Jessie and three of her sisters, Arabelle, Carrie, and Ella. The oldest daughter, Emma, had married Leonard Patchen in Oswego, New York, in 1868. It seems likely that between 1872 and 1874 Leonard and Emma moved to Minnesota, where five of their seven children were born, and that Laurena Haskins, with her four younger daughters, followed them. Arabelle married Marshall Williams in St. Paul in December 1874 and moved to Stevens County in western Minnesota. In 1886 there were two more marriages. Ella married Arthur

My own dear wife. I now sit down in lownliness to write a few lines to my wife and children. I am lonely tho I need not tell you that for you know it by experiance. . . .

My dear wife you no that it is three years since I took a pen in my hand to write before. You must excuse my writing for it comes from a pure hand and heart. Kiss my babes for me.

Letter, Hiram Haskins to Laurena Haskins, 1857

My own dear wife. I received a kind letter from you today and hastin to ansur it for I know you air anxus to here from me. We are on our way for some wheres. John was here just now with the last load. I am well but not very tough. We take a steemer for God knows where but I will write soon again thrue Cap McKinley. Day before yesterday I was promoted to corprell and today lutenant. McKinley is well. Go and tell mister Rathburn John is well. Mc gave me a sword and belt. John went to New Orleans this after noon and got my fitout. You must bory money of some one for this money I will have to use but I will write soon. Give my love to all who may inquire. Tell my children they must be good. A kiss for you all from your kind Husband.

Letter, Hiram Haskins to Laurena Haskins, 1863

Holly, and eventually they moved west to Spokane, Washington. Carrie married Clinton Backus and stayed in St. Paul.[9] Carrie and Clinton were well-known educators in the St. Paul community. Clinton conducted the Baldwin Seminary[10] and Carrie later operated Oak Hill, a school which educated the daughters of many prominent St. Paul citizens.[11]

In September 1883 Jessie was enrolled as a boarding student in the academy at Carleton. Among her classmates was Michael Dowling, who was a remarkable young man.[12] Born in February 1866, he was the son of John and Honora Dowling of Huntington, Massachusetts. Michael moved to St. Louis with his father after his mother's death in 1876. After a brief move to Chicago, Michael left his father and moved to Minnesota on his own. He worked as a farmhand and cattle herder in Canby, and there his life would be changed dramatically. In December 1881 while tending cattle, Dowling was trapped in a severe blizzard and suffered frostbite that resulted in the amputation of both his legs below the knee, one arm below the elbow, and most of the fingers of the other hand. He became a ward of the state and lived in a foster home for most of the next two years. In 1883 Dowling proposed to the Yellow Medicine Board of County Commissioners that if they supplied him with artificial limbs and tuition for two terms at Carleton, he would make no future claims on the county.

The commissioners agreed, and Michael Dowling joined Jessie Haskins in the new class that arrived at Carleton in September 1883. Dowling's self-assurance and confidence in the face of his new disability, and his subsequent success in life as an editor and politician must have influenced Jessie.[13]

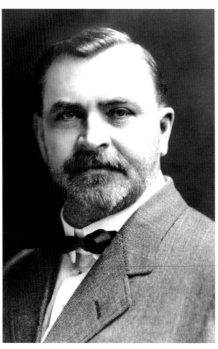

Michael J. Dowling, circa 1920

Jessie remained in the academy at Carleton for two years. During that time her mother briefly moved to Herman, Minnesota, then returned to St. Paul where the family took up residence at 550 DeBow Street. It is not known why Jessie failed to continue on into college at Carleton. A probable reason was money. Jessie's mother moved again, this time to Kettle Falls, Washington, and there the family seems to have prospered because Jessie planned to return to

Carleton and complete her education. In 1891, at the age of twenty-five, she was injured in a fall from a horse while on an outing near the Columbia River in Kettle Falls. The horse reared back, fell, and probably rolled over on her. She had several rib fractures, and her shoulder was broken in three places. The shoulder healed imperfectly, and the deformity accentuated her spine curvature. It was a year before she recovered enough to care for herself or was even able to raise her hands to her hair. Her recovery included travel to Boston for treatment. By 1895 she was ready to return to Carleton.[14]

The Carleton College catalogue for 1895-96 listed Jessie as a freshman. Her class schedule was challenging, including Latin, German, mathematics, the Bible, the Iliad, and history in the fall session. The return to such a rigorous academic environment at the age of twenty-nine, after a recent serious injury and rehabilitation, must have been difficult. Jessie's grades that first term were B, C, D, C-, C, and D. Her record also includes seven days of unexcused absence, perhaps days spent with Carrie and her husband in St. Paul. The situation did not improve much in the winter and spring sessions. Jessie reduced the number of her classes, but over those two terms she received four C's, three D's, and dropped out of another class before completing the work. The results altered her academic standing.[15] The Carleton catalogue for 1896–97 listed her as a student in Special Courses, not a candidate for a degree.

Class studies weren't Jessie's only interest. On October 12, 1895, the Gamma Delta Society elected her a member. Gamma Delta members, all women students, conducted monthly literary sessions that included student essays, "conversationals" or talks on some topic, and debates. The society was well run and disciplined. The officers met each month to create agendas and supervise the membership. They seemed to appreciate timeliness at their literary sessions for they refused to grant Jessie an excuse for being tardy at the December session. The society encouraged debate, discussion, and friendship, and developed skills of critical thinking in its members.

Jessie's skills as a public speaker became evident at Gamma Delta meetings. Debates were structured in traditional style: a statement was put forth, and a student or two was appointed to speak in support of, or against, the statement.

In three years Jessie participated in seventeen debates which included the following statements (with the position she defended):

Is the calling of the physician as great a power for good as that of a clergyman? (yes)

Is the University science course more beneficial to the nation than the classical course? (no)

Should law always be enforced? (yes)

Are the persecutions of the Jews in Russia justifiable and warrantable? (no)

Has the optimism of Dickens directed society more than the pessimism of Thackeray? (no)

Is Christianity impossible without a church and a creed? (no)

Ought we to expect in America the same care for city streets as is shown in European cities? (no)

Do modern cities have as great a power on our society and civilization as ancient cities? (no)

Shall we have free coinage of silver in the United States? (yes)

Should John Brown be regarded as a hero and martyr rather than a fanatic? (yes)

Are fraternities against literary societies? (yes)

The hope of the general federation of women's clubs to secure systematic instruction in morals in the public schools is well-founded. (yes)

Was Governor Clough justified in vetoing the Forest Warden's bill? (no)

Is it in the interests of civilization for England to gain control of South Africa? (yes)

Is the influence of the fine arts favorable to religion? (yes)

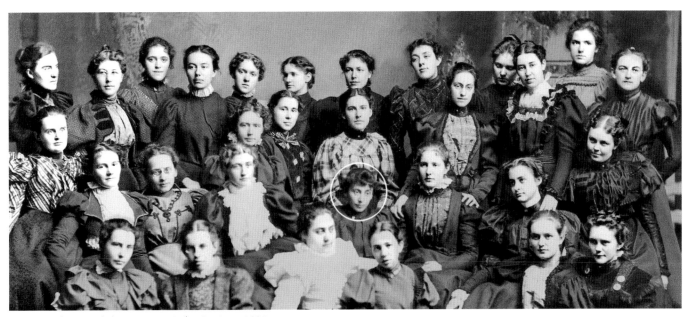

Jessie Haskins and the Gamma Delta Society, 1898

Jessie or her side won fourteen of these debates, lost two, and received a tie decision in the other. Jessie also gave several orations on such topics as the prize system in English universities, Seventh Day Adventists, poet Alfred Austin, snowstorms, and Rudyard Kipling's notion of women.[16]

Most of these presentations were ahead of her in 1896 when she received a response to this January 27th letter to the editor of the Minnesota Bulletin of Corrections and Charities, published at the State Capitol.

Sir: It seems as though something should be done to provide schools for deformed and crippled children. Though we have institutions for the blind and deaf, this other class of children are left to attend the public schools at which they study the same hours, and in every way contend with strong, well children as best they may. In the past years great progress has been made in Europe in treating cases of spinal disease, hip disease, and similar diseases, but for only the last seven or eight years have such cases been treated successfully in this country, and this only in two or three of our large cities. Poor parents, or even people of moderate means, in our Western States, are not able to have such children treated properly; in fact, it is almost impossible for them to learn that anything can be done for such children. And so children that could have been easily cured at first, grow up uncared for, and gradually grow worse and worse until they are incurable. Many cases of spinal curvature, for instance, develop slowly, and are almost unnoticed until the child reaches the age of twelve or fourteen. A great many such children are in our public schools, uncared for and constantly sitting in positions and doing tasks at which they grow worse. Surely these children have a right to have proper schools provided for them. We should have state institutions where these children could have the latest scientific treatment and their education could progress under more favorable circumstances than in the public schools. The expense of such an institution to the state would not be as great accordingly as the institutions for the education of other defective children, for the best authorities on such cases agree that hundreds of cases, if taken in time and given systematic treatment such as it is impossible to give in homes, would be cured speedily.

J.A.H.

As a result, Jessie was invited to speak to the Fifth Minnesota State Conference of Corrections and Charities, held at Red Wing on November 17–19. Her paper, "The Need of an Institution for

Crippled and Deformed Children," was one of twenty-four presented at the conference, which was attend-ed by more than 100 dele-gates. Also on the program was a paper by Pearson on "Altruism and Reform." The combination of the two presentations supports the belief that Pearson had become an important advisor to Jessie in her desire to help crippled children and that Pearson had used his friendship with Hastings Hart to help Jessie. Hart must have seen sincerity and merit in her plea for help and pushed the organizing committee into placing her on the program.

In fact, Jessie considered refus-ing the invitation of the Board of Corrections and Charities to speak in Red Wing. She told Ella, by then married and living in Spokane, of her reluctance to participate in the conference. Ella later wrote: "I immediately replied impulsively, and without much realization of the mental anguish which these speech-es must cause her, that 'if she thought she could do something for those poor little things and did not, she should be ashamed of herself.' She told me afterward that when she felt something was too hard to attempt she would spur herself on with the thought, 'if you can't do it for those little things you should be ashamed of yourself.' So you can see it was not easy for her to do."

Jessie's paper followed the basic logic outlined in her original letter, which called for crippled children to receive, as a basic right, an education appropriate to their condition. This time Jessie point-ed out the benefit of such an education to the state:

Take a child, for instance, with hip disease. Often the treatment is long and painful, but there is no reason the mind should not be trained. These children above all others need mental equipment for the life work which will in time surely press upon them. There are many employments that such children could be trained for with profit to themselves and to the state, and yet they often waste their childhood uncared for, untrained, and drag out a weary life contending with problems for which their stronger brothers and sisters have had ample training. It seems as though the justice of this measure must speak for itself. Surely it is best for the state that such children should be cured whenever possible, and educated so that they may be helpful, self-sustaining members of the state.

Her paper also called for the best possible medical care at the institution. A crucial expansion had developed in Jessie's argu-ment: the care of crippled children was more than a gift to a special interest group. It was also good public policy.[17]

The conference received extensive coverage in the Red Wing, St. Paul, and Minneapolis newspapers.[18] The conference minutes include some of the discussion sessions, but the extent of the response to Jessie's presen-tation is unknown. Jessie asked the Board of Corrections and

It was a very hard winter and there was much suffering among the poor of the large cities.

My sister was deeply moved by the incident.

My sister said that the hardest thing to combat was the belief that nothing could be done unless at some indefinite time in the future, while she wanted to do something at once.

What it was for my sister to appear before these committees and others you can perhaps judge from what I have said of our reticence in the family of even mentioning the matter of her misfortune to her, and now she was called upon to appear before strangers and make a plea for these children for the help they needed, using her own experience as an instance of what these poor little things could be saved from.

That her plea was moving I know, as she was an eloquent speaker, and the fact that she gained not only the attention but the aid of the people whom she addressed, proves it.

Ella (Haskins) Holly
Spokane, 1945

Charities to create an institution along the lines she had discussed, but was told that such an effort was beyond the scope of the board's ability. Most likely it was Hastings Hart who conceived the notion of approaching the state legislature, and most likely it was Hastings Hart who brought Jessie Haskins and Arthur Gillette together.[19]

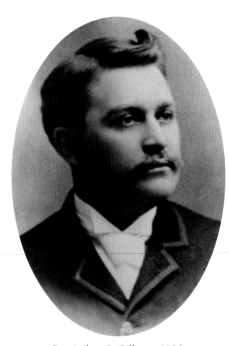

Dr. Arthur J. Gillette, 1896

Arthur Jay Gillette was born at Prairieville, in Rice County, Minnesota, on October 28, 1864, to Albert and Ellen (Austin) Gillette. Soon after his birth the family moved to a farm close to South St. Paul on land that became part of the site of the city's stockyards. Arthur attended country schools until he was old enough for more formal education. His father didn't support his desire to leave home for more formal education, but his mother interceded, pointing out that

Arthur really wasn't cut out to be a farmer, and his father agreed. Arthur attended Hamline University from 1880 to 1883 and then entered Minnesota Hospital College of Medicine, where he studied until it closed in 1885. He then transferred to the reorganized St. Paul Medical College for a year of study, graduating in 1886.

After a brief internship at St. Joseph's Hospital in St. Paul, Gillette went to New York City in late 1886 to study orthopaedic medicine with Lewis Sayer. At that time Sayer was a preeminent American orthopaedist, having published *Lectures on Orthopaedic Surgery and Diseases of the Joint* in 1876. Sayer had devised sur-geries for clubfoot and tuberculosis of the hip and introduced a plaster of Paris jacket for the treatment of Pott's disease and scoliosis (curvature of the spine). Gillette spent a second year in New York as a house surgeon at the New York Orthopaedic Dispensary and Hospital. There he studied orthopaedics with Newton Shaffer, an equal and peer of Sayer's and chairman of orthopaedics at Cornell Medical School. Shaffer stressed patient and conscientious application of mechanical and therapeutic techniques to achieve correction of deformities, including traction, bracing, and physical exercise.[20]

These two years had a profound effect on Gillette. He returned to St. Paul in 1888 with great expectations, hoping to bring his new knowledge home to a waiting community. He found little encouragement. Looking

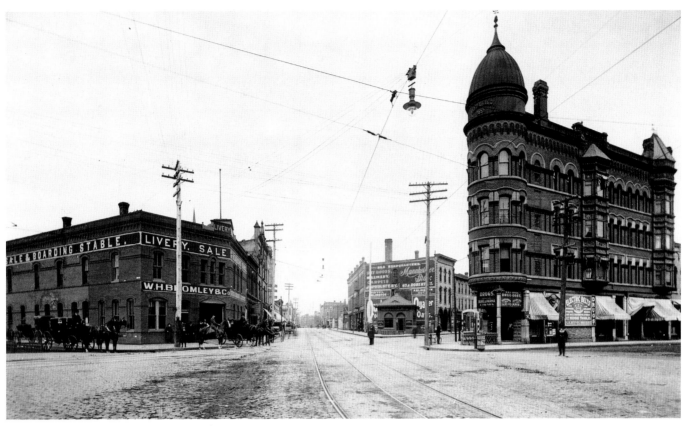

Seven Corners, St. Paul, circa 1902–1904

back he said in 1916: "Well do I remember, when I consulted a few of my medical teachers and asked them what they thought of my taking up orthopaedic surgery in Minnesota. They said, 'It is very nice work if you like it, but you cannot possibly make a living from it for there are not enough cases, and then too, when deformities do develop they always seem to thrive in a poor family.'"[21]

Instead Gillette opened a general medical practice office in the Seven Corners area of St. Paul and took up residence nearby on Pleasant Avenue. Gradually he began to see more and more people with orthopaedic problems, including crippled children. By 1890 he felt secure enough to devote his practice exclusively to orthopaedics,

and he became the first full-time orthopaedist in Minnesota.

Gillette was not the only Minnesota physician with an interest in orthopaedics. Dr. A. B. Stewart of Winona published an article in the *Northwestern Medical and Surgical Journal* in 1871 describing his experience in dividing tendons to correct deformities.[22] In 1875 the Minnesota Orthopedic Institute was formed in St. Paul to manufacture and sell orthopaedic appliances to correct deformities. From 1879 to his death in 1909, Dr. Ernest Horst cared for a significant number of orthopaedic patients in his practice in St. Paul. In 1887 Dr. James E. Moore, later a giant figure at the University of Minnesota Medical School, published a text on

orthopaedic surgery after he returned to Minnesota from studying in New York, London,

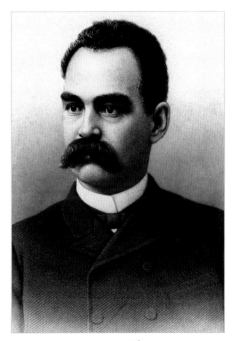

Dr. James E. Moore, 1896

and Berlin. Moore was professor of orthopaedics, as well as surgery, at both the Minnesota Hospital College and the St. Paul Medical College until those schools gave up their charters in favor of the new medical school at the University of Minnesota.[23]

While not alone in his interest in orthopaedic problems, Arthur Gillette quickly set himself apart in his dedication to the specialty. He soon became the orthopaedic surgeon for St. Joseph's, St. Luke's, Bethesda, and City and County hospitals in St. Paul, and was a prolific speaker and writer. Some of his early publications, which reached local and national audiences, included:

> *Bowed Leg—Combined Osteotomy and Osteoclasis* (1890)
>
> *The Simplest and Most Rational Treatment of Club Foot* (1890)
>
> *Rachitis and Resulting Deformities* (1890)
>
> *Orthopedic Surgery as a Specialty* (1891)
>
> *Pott's Disease with Special Reference to Treatment in the Upper Dorsal and Cervical Regions* (1892)
>
> *Two Cases of Tuberculous Knee Joint Disease* (1892)
>
> *Mechanical and Forcible Straightening of Old Deformities of the Knee Joint* (1895)
>
> *Sprains* (1897)
>
> *Traumatic Spondylitis* (1897)

Many more were to follow.[24] Gillette was a member of a large number of medical societies and civic groups, where he was

routinely well-liked and highly regarded. It is impossible, in numerous and diverse sources, to find a negative or even ambivalent comment about him. He developed a reputation for a special interest in children, and in his publications and correspondence Gillette made pointed observations about some of the children he treated. He noticed that most crippling conditions flourished among the poor, and that poor children could not receive effective treatment and proper care. He believed that few physicians had sufficient knowledge or skill to treat such children adequately. He described some of the prevailing attitudes toward children with deformities. Many parents at that time, he noted, considered a deformed child a family disgrace and concealed the child, creating the notion that children with deformities were rare or the result of some family disease or horrible mental impression the mother experienced in pregnancy. While some children were secluded out of pity, many were hidden away so that their deformities might not frighten another pregnant woman and create yet another deformed child.[25]

Gillette treated many children without charge and even paid the hospital costs of several who were under his care. This behavior could not have gone unnoticed by Hastings Hart, whose office was in St. Paul and whose charity work certainly included some of the people Gillette saw as patients. It appears that Hart sent Jessie

Haskins to see Gillette in the six weeks between the November 1896 conference in Red Wing and the opening of the legislative session in January 1897. Gillette described the visit later:

It came about in this way. . . . Just before the meeting of the last legislature a young lady came into my office. I noticed that she was somewhat deformed, and naturally supposed that she came to consult me in my professional capacity. She soon explained, however, that she did not come to see me about herself, though she said she supposed her deformity had been noticed. She gave every evidence of being a lady, and I was soon greatly interested in her suggestion. She wanted to know if I would be interested in a state institution for crippled and deformed children. She informed me that her name was Jessie Haskins and that she was connected with Carleton College. Her permanent deformity, she said, was due to neglect in childhood, when it might have been remedied. Her parents had traveled with her from state to state seeking some cure or relief, but in vain. Her sufferings and her understanding of the sorrows of crippled people naturally aroused her sympathy with all the crippled and deformed, and suggested to her the necessity of doing something for the deformed children of the poor. Who could do such a work better than the state? I told Miss Haskins at once that I was in sympathy with her undertaking.[26]

The bill that was introduced in the legislature was written by Hart, and it is extremely unlikely that he would have sought sponsorship of the bill without counsel and substantial support from someone besides Jessie Haskins. By sending Jessie to Arthur Gillette, he linked passion with

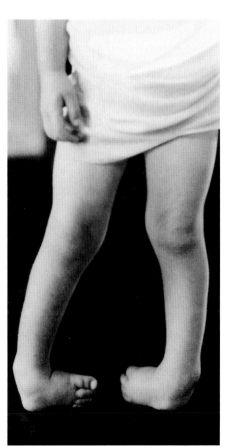
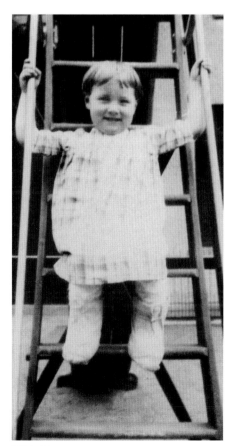
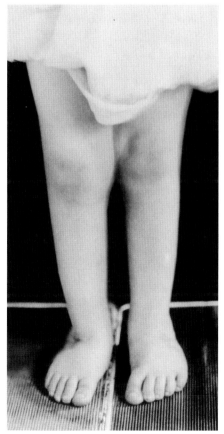

Verna Pratt with club feet and her treatment, 1921–23

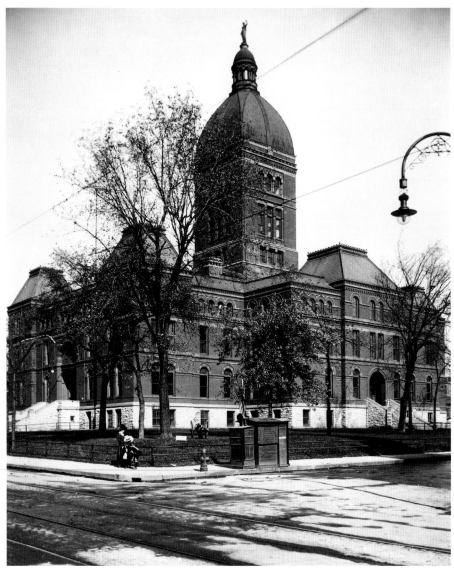

State Capitol, St. Paul, Minnesota, circa 1900

political party. This was amended to a board of five persons appointed by the governor; at least three were to be women. The committee recommended that five thousand dollars be appropriated each year for two years. The bill was printed and sent to the Senate on the seventy-seventh day. There its progress stopped abruptly.[27]

The session was in its final days, and committees were overwhelmed with work. The hospital bill almost died in the Senate Committee on Finance. Its supporters turned to the community, and a lengthy supportive article appeared in the *Saint Paul Pioneer Press* on April 7. It leaned heavily on Jessie Haskins's presentation in Red Wing, which had been published with the conference proceedings in March. The writer also included quotes from Jessie's appeals to legislative committees. Additional support came from the Northfield newspapers. In editorials the papers acknowledged the state's tight finances during the national depression that started in 1893, but argued that balancing the budget should not be done at the expense of the unfortunate. The publicity seemed to have no effect. In the end, a chance encounter proved to be more important than logic.[28]

A senator from southern Minnesota was adamantly opposed to the bill, and it was thought important for Jessie to speak to him. Jessie boarded a train in Northfield, prepared to make yet another appeal in

experience and devised an effective team to bring the message to the politicians.

Hart's bill, described as an act to establish a "Minnesota Institute for Crippled and Deformed Children," was introduced as House File 749 by Representative Duren F. Kelley of Northfield on the forty-seventh day of the legislative session. The bill was referred to the Committee on General Legislation. There it was amended to include a requirement that care be provided at an institution within ten miles of the University of Minnesota. The bill went to the Committee on Appropriations on the sixty-eighth day of the session and was amended again due to some disagreement over governance structure. The original governing board of the new institution was designed along the lines of the Board of Corrections and Charities: six persons, with no more than three from one

St. Paul. Two men took a seat just in front of her. Overhearing their conversation, Jessie learned that one of them was a legislator. Ella (Haskins) Holly explained what Jessie did next.

When his companion left him, she leaned forward and asked if she might speak to him as she saw he was a member of the legislature and she wished to get in touch with as many members as possible as she was going up to see a committee about a bill in which she was interested. She said that he appeared to be a little amused, but was very courteous and willing to listen. She told him it was the bill for a state hospital for crippled children, and his face immediately hardened. He said quickly, "I am opposed to that bill. I shall vote against it if it comes up." She said to him, "Why?" She said he looked at her for a moment, and then he said harshly, "because I will not let those children be taken to a State Hospital to be experimented on by doctors!"

Jessie told Ella that she explained Dr. Gillette's work, and how the place was to be run. Ella described the appeal that Jessie made to the senator:

She laid bare her young sensitive soul and the unhappiness which her misfortune had given her. He listened, and

before they reached St. Paul he told her that he had never viewed it in that light before, and that he would talk to Dr. Gillette and see if anything could be done. She said that she believed that it was Divine Providence which brought about that meeting, for it was Senator A. W. Stockton of Faribault, and he not only withdrew his opposition to the bill, but became active in pushing it and ended by rescuing it from the oblivion of the committee room.[29]

The serendipity of this meeting was followed by Arthur Gillette's appearance before the Committee on Finance. An article describing Dr. Gillette's meeting with the committee was subsequently published in the *Minneapolis Journal.*

I went before the committee and, while I found them kind and courteous, they informed me that they did not believe it would be possible to pass a bill for such a hospital in the face of the existing hard times. However, they were

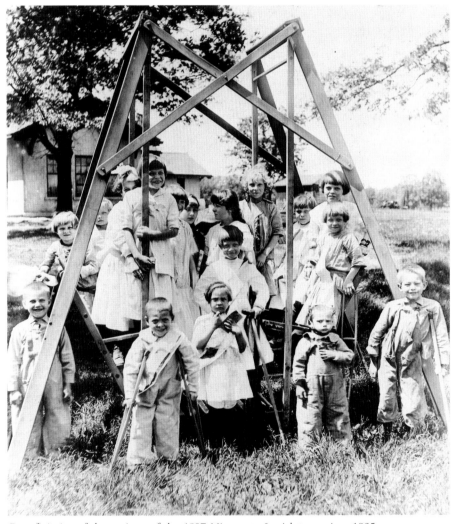

Beneficiaries of the actions of the 1897 Minnesota Legislature, circa 1925

kind enough to listen to what I had to say. Then, in the natural practical way of business men, they asked very pertinent questions, which showed that they were taking an interest in the matter. Where were they to be cared for was one question. It was pointed out that in either St. Paul or Minneapolis there were hospitals which were well equipped for such work and that it would not be necessary at first to build a separate hospital for the work, as they had thought. Then they asked: what would be the price a competent man would demand to take charge of the surgical work? They were assured that doctors could be found in either city who would be glad to take care of the little unfortunates without charge if the state would furnish the money for their hospital expenses and the necessary surgical instruments and appliances. It seemed that this information struck the keynote. For the first time the committee began to realize that it was not a money making or political scheme of any sort.[30]

Gillette's personal commitment to find physicians to provide free care, and perhaps his stature as president of the Ramsey County Medical Society, won over the skeptics, but the issue of governance still bothered the committee members. The *Minneapolis Journal* described Gillette's response. "Then arose the question: who should have charge of the administration of the appropriation? In my desperation to think of someone who would have no other interest than that of helping the poor cripples I suggested the regents of the state university, in whom everybody has confidence."[31] Gillette's impromptu idea was taken seriously. The Senate amended the bill to remove the public governing board and made the university regents responsible for the care and treatment of the children. On April 23, 1897, the eighty-third and last day of the session, the bill was passed unanimously by the Senate. That evening Representative Kelley, the original sponsor, moved that the House accept the bill as amended by the Senate. It was approved 88 to 2 in the last moments of the session and published as Chapter 289 of the laws of 1897.[32]

After his experience with the Senate, Gillette was unsure the bill would pass. The *Minneapolis Journal* reported his concern: "You can imagine my surprise when I found that the bill had passed, and that it was one of the last that had got by the legislature. But Miss Haskins had stuck by the bill to the end and stayed around the capitol and battled for it till it passed."[33] Jessie spent those last hours at the Capitol on a bench outside the House chamber with Carrie and Clinton Backus.

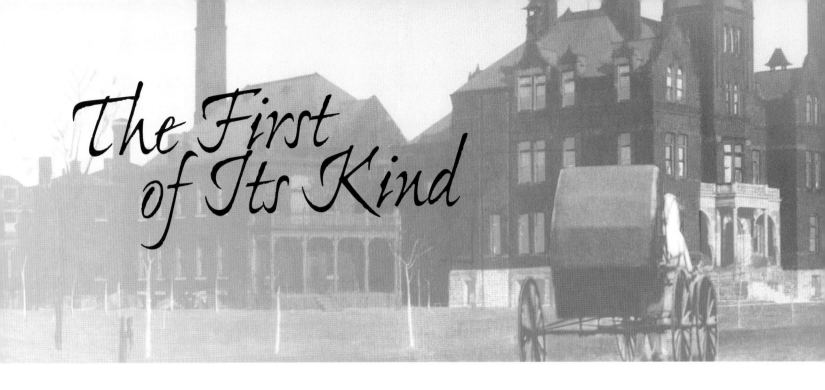

The First of Its Kind

Whatever its surprise at being required to supervise the care and treatment of crippled children, the University of Minnesota's Board of Regents responded quickly to the task. A new hospital for crippled children had been created, but the legislature did not want new buildings. Instead, the children were to receive care in space available in one of the institutions in Minneapolis or St. Paul, a sort of hospital within a hospital.

A subcommittee of the board, consisting of regents Stephen Mahoney, Greenleaf Clark, and Mylo Todd, met in the summer months of 1897 to select a host institution and formulate the rules and regulations for governing the new crippled children's hospital. Their guidelines fell into four broad areas: admission criteria, medical care, medical records, and a provision to allow the executive committee of the regents to act for the entire board.[1]

Any interested person could request admission to the hospital. That person was required to complete an affidavit that included the child's name, age, and address, as well as those of the child's parents, a statement of the length of time the child had lived in Minnesota, the occupation and property of the parents, and whether they possessed the means to obtain medical care for the child. A physician was required to examine the child and document the health problem. If the family attended a church, a statement was required from their clergyman attesting to their inability to obtain medical care for their child. The entire application was forwarded to the board of regents, which consulted with its own physician and determined whether the child should receive care at the newly-designated State Hospital for Crippled and Deformed Children.[2]

The regents stipulated that only children between the ages of two and twelve years at the time of the initial application could receive care at the hospital, and only if they had lived in Minnesota for at least a year. Their parents were responsible for transportation to and from the hospital and also were required to provide all the clothing their child would need during the hospital stay. Braces and appliances supplied to the child remained the property of the state.

Children were to be discharged when they were cured, when no benefit could be found with further treatment, or if their original diagnosis was found to be wrong and the new diagnosis was inappropriate for care at the hospital.[3]

The specific rules and regulations were approved at the regents' meeting of August 25, 1897. They established a surgeon-in-chief position, a supervising physician who would have "full control" over the hospital's daily affairs. Arthur Gillette was appointed to the post without pay. The university's medical school was required to provide other physicians as needed, and as a result Dr. James Moore was named consulting physician and surgeon. The regents also defined the criteria for selecting an institution to house the new hospital. The host institution was required to provide a ward to be used exclusively for the care of the children, provide support services equivalent to those given to other patients, and help maintain a separate medical record for each child. That record was to include the child's name and address, admission and discharge dates, diagnoses, surgeries, treatment, and final outcome. A formal report, summarizing the work of the hospital, was to be given to the regents annually.

During that August meeting Mahoney, Clark, and Todd also recommended that the City and County Hospital in St. Paul be chosen as the site for the new hospital. The committee had solicited proposals from hospitals in Minneapolis and St. Paul and visit-

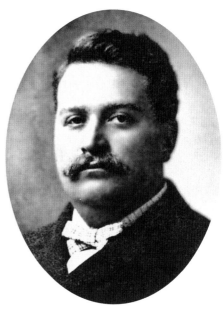

Dr. Arthur J. Gillette, 1902

ed several of them. They listed the best hospitals as City and County Hospital, St. Luke's and St. Joseph's in St. Paul, and St. Barnabas and St. Mary's in Minneapolis (there was no hospital at the University of Minnesota at the time). The board of regents accepted City and County Hospital's bid and directed that a two-year contract be drawn up. Anticipating the need to supervise the affairs of the new hospital, as well as the medical school of the university, the regents organized four standing committees of the board: Executive, Agriculture, Medical, and Law.[4]

City and County Hospital was a public facility located off West Seventh Street and was supervised by the Ramsey County Board of Control. Its superintendent, Dr. Arthur Ancker, was an energetic, demanding, and strong-willed man whose hard work resulted in recognition of the hospital as one of the best in the region. The medical staff included

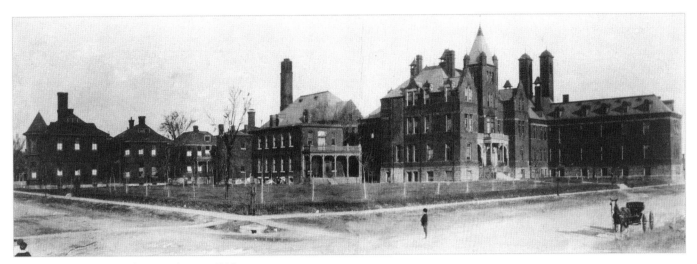

City and County Hospital, St. Paul, circa 1899

Arthur Gillette as orthopaedic surgeon, and Perry Millard and Parks Ritchie, future deans of the university's medical school. In 1897 there were 1,532 admissions and an average daily census of 125 patients. The hospital spent $30,657 on patient care, or $4.70 per patient per week. Electricity and a new boiler were installed that year at a cost of $5,461. Dr. Ancker's salary was $3,500.[5]

While the search for a host hospital appears to have been an open process, the regents clearly looked to Arthur Gillette for guidance. Beyond his demonstrated commitment to children with deformities, his stature was enhanced by the recommendation of the executive committee of the medical school's faculty that he be promoted from instructor to professor of orthopaedic surgery.[6] In his appearance before the legislature he had volunteered to provide free care for the children from the medical profession. Certainly the regents chose a good host hospital, but they also chose a hospital that was convenient for Dr. Gillette, whose office and home were in St. Paul. Dr. Ancker played his part, too. Gillette recalled years later that Ancker was so anxious to have the hospital that he told the search committee that if they would tell him the bids of the other hospitals, he would "go them one better." City and County Hospital's bid of $3.75 per week for children under twelve years of age, and $4.50 per week for children aged twelve to sixteen years of age, was 25 cents

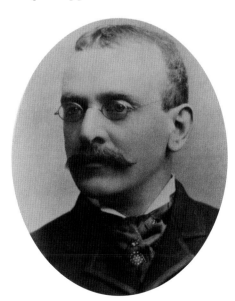

Dr. Arthur B. Ancker, 1894

I find a discarded splint which belongs to us which by making a few changes costing about $2.00 would fit her exactly. A patient who had club foot is so nearly well that by applying a specially made leather support he could go home the cost of which will not exceed $1.50. If you will order it I will have these braces repaired.

**Dr. Arthur Gillette
to Stephen Mahoney, 1902**

He is undoubtedly an idiot and any small thing we could do to cure the deformity in his foot would not be of any avail.

**Dr. Wallace Cole
to State Board of Control, 1915**

The child's tuberculosis of the spine and hips had caused a severe deformity of the spine and tightening of the muscles of the hip. He also was in poor health from his long fight with tuberculosis.

The hospital treatment lasted 536 days. The boy's draining sores were dressed, and his tight hip muscles were overcome with traction and weights. His spine deformity was improved with a plaster of Paris body cast. With good nutrition and a clean, healthy environment, his tuberculosis disappeared. Gillette was proud of the result: "Today, without causing him one bit of pain or suffering, all of these sinuses are healed, he is almost perfectly straight, and is running about the [hospital] campus with bat and ball, a pleasure he has never known before."[8]

The result stood the test of time. Writing to the hospital in 1920, Royal Gray, by then a young man, gave proof of the value of his treatment, not without a sense of humor:

Letter requesting admission of first patient, 1897

lower per week per child than that of the closest competitor.[7]

The first admission occurred on October 27, 1897, at 8:45 in the morning. The child was Royal Gray, a ten-year-old boy from Pine City who had contracted tuberculosis five years earlier. Dr. Gillette carefully documented the boy's story in his first report to the board of regents:

Our first patient was a little boy from a country district. His parents had spent what little money they could get together from time to time for treatment and apparatus, but the treatment was so interrupted owing to the lack of funds that the few dollars they spent in this direction were wasted, and he came to us unable to walk—almost bent double by the deformity of the back and contraction of the muscles. He had seven draining sinuses.

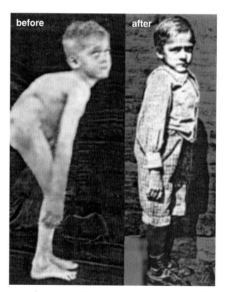

Royal J. Gray, first patient admitted, 1897

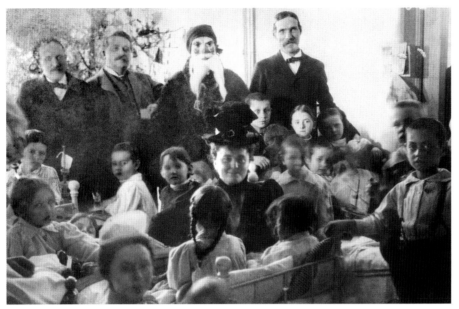

Dr. Ancker, Dr. Gillette, Judge Mahoney, and the children at Christmas, 1899

Well, it has been a long time since I left there. Nevertheless I have often thought of the time I spent with you all. Well, to begin with, I went to school after I left the hospital until I was 19 years old. I then started working for myself doing such things as painting, carrying mail on a 27 mile route out of Pine City, and then to the automobile game and have been at it ever since. At present I am running a taxi business of my own in Virginia, Minnesota, and am doing pretty good considering the high cost of everything. And as to my health I have never had a doctor since I left the hospital and am in the best of health at present. But the worst of all is I have become a victim of a woman, and we were married September 20, 1915, and have two children.

As for his doctor, "I sure have lots of praise for Dr. Gillette and have told people about him all over the country."[9]

By the end of 1898, thirty-five applications for admission had been received. Eleven were denied, although four patients received limited care without admission to the hospital. Of the twenty-four approved applications, eleven children had tuberculosis, six had clubfoot, two had dislocations of the hip, two had cerebral palsy, and the remaining three had other conditions. The first annual report to the regents described all but three of the children as cured or improved as result of their treatment. One child was removed by his parents before treatment was complete. One died from a sudden intestinal illness. A third child, diagnosed with cerebral palsy, was "pronounced an idiot and incurable." The regents spent $2,147.82 of the $5,000 allowed by the legislature for the first year of operations.[10]

Your letter of yesterday is at hand. If the mother of the child would find a place to board near the hospital in St. Paul, I presume there would be no objection to having her come to the hospital every day and see the child if she desired to do so. She could not board in the hospital and her services would not be needed as a nurse for there are plenty of nurses to take care of the children.

**Stephen Mahoney
to a family, 1898**

I am feeling very blue today as you know we lost a little boy in the State ward yesterday dying from tuberculosis of the lungs and other internal organs. For the past two or three days another little boy at the hospital has been very ill from an abscess in his head, probably tuberculosis, and I am afraid he cannot live. While this is bound to occur frequently in handling such tuberculous children, yet it makes me feel very badly when it does occur.

**Dr. Arthur Gillette
to Stephen Mahoney, 1904**

The process of applying for care for a child brought about a close relationship between Arthur Gillette and Stephen Mahoney, who was one of sixteen students to graduate from the University of Minnesota in 1877. He subsequently obtained a law degree from the University of Michigan and served as a Minneapolis municipal court judge for twelve years. He became, in 1889, the first Minnesota alumnus to serve as a regent.[11] Because the approval of the board of regents was required for care at the hospital, Gillette and Mahoney corresponded regarding virtually every application received between 1897 and 1907. They genuinely liked each other and became friends. They approved the application of any child whose needs met the legal criteria and found ways to provide care for many other children who were "special cases." These were children who were older or younger than the established age limits, or children whose parents could afford to pay for some medical care but not the long hospital stay required to change their crippling condition. The emphasis remained on poor children with deformities that could be improved with care, meaning that they could be expected to become self-sufficient. The applications of some children were denied because their condition was deemed hopeless. Others were turned away because they were "cretins, idiots, or morons." These terms, not used today, were common at the time and described mentally incompe-

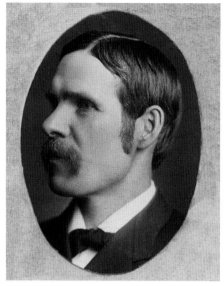

Judge Stephen Mahoney, circa 1905

tent children who were unlikely to become independent, self-supporting citizens.[12]

Despite the successes, referrals came slowly. Dr. Gillette made a presentation to the Sixth Minnesota Conference of Charities and Corrections, held in St. Cloud in November 1897. His talk, "The Duty of the State to its Indigent Cripple Children," outlined the principles of care for children with deformities.[13] The *Minneapolis Journal* provided publicity in an extensive article on August 6, 1898. The journalist accompanied Dr. Gillette during a day's work at the hospital, and his description must have gone a long way towards dispelling the widespread fear of hospitals:

> [I was] amazed to find [the hospital] beautifully situated overlooking the Mississippi River. The buildings are substantial and imposing and rise from a spacious green lawn, kept in the best of

order. Inside everything is arranged with consideration for economy of time and effort. Everything is spotlessly clean from the basement to the roof. The hospital is itself encouragement for the sick and wounded to get well. It is a palace compared to the barn that does service for a city hospital in Minneapolis. There is a perfect system of ventilation, and one smells none of those vile odors compounded of sewage smells and kitchen effluvia that are so nauseating in some so-called hospitals.

The writer gave an attractive account of the children's daily routine. "All of the patients who are not confined to their beds are given the free run of the big hospital lawn, and there on a bright day they may be seen hobbling and limping around at their games, quite as happy as more fortunate children. . . . Instead of shrieks of pain and moans of anguish there were peals of joyous childish laughter. Instead of drawn pallid faces there were red-cheeked, jolly, fat faces and sparkling eyes."

The writer also gave a glimpse of Dr. Gillette's relationship with the children. "Though the children are perfectly happy and well it is a great joke with them to ask the doctor every day when they can go home. As he leaves the ward most of them limp or hobble to the door and call out 'say Doc, when can I go home?' 'Right away,' answers the doctor, and the little fellows laugh."[14]

The regents were pleased. In the hospital's first annual report to the legislature, they said: "If these children are taken while young they may be saved from the terrible misfortune of going through life cripples and hunchbacks. Instead of being helpless paupers and beggars, they become respectable, self-support-

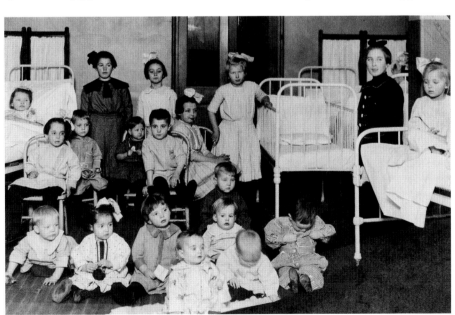

Children in the ward, circa 1905

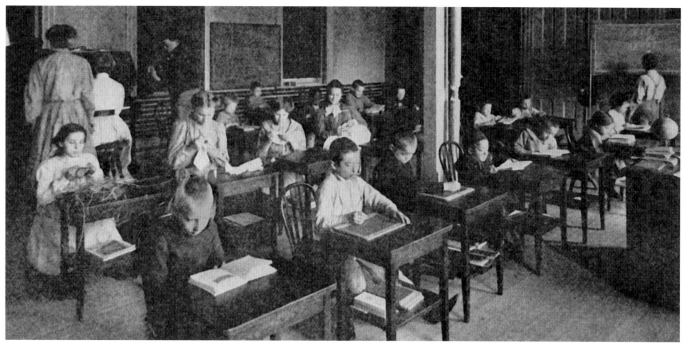

The schoolroom, circa 1900

ing citizens." The regents had not been consulted when the legislature created the hospital in 1897, but despite being given the unexpected task of supervising the hospital, they were convinced of the merit of the work. Their report includes their opinion of the hospital: "It is difficult to imagine a more humane or a more profitable work in which the state could engage or to which it could devote a small part of its revenue." And, they made special note of Dr. Gillette: "So enthusiastic and devoted has he been to these poor children . . . that no private patients in any hospital have had better care and attention." However, the regents were uncomfortable supervising the hospital. The report closed with a request:

> The work of carrying out the provisions of the law . . . is entirely foreign to the duties of the Board of Regents in the management of the University. The legislature saw fit to assign to the Board the duty of inaugurating and carrying on the work for two years. We have made an earnest effort to give it a fair trial . . . and if the legis-lature, at its coming session, shall be able to find some other agency through which the state can carry on this work we shall be much pleased.

It would be a decade before their plea was answered.[15]

Jessie Haskins's original plea for good education for children with deformities was not forgotten. In 1898 Dr. Gillette employed a school teacher, Frances Boardman, at a salary of $35 per month to provide "such instruction as they are capable of receiving." The children's schoolwork was balanced by drawing, sewing, stories, and singing. A piano was placed on the ward, and keeping it clean became a source of pride for the older children. The curriculum grew until lessons were given at every level through eighth grade. Miss Boardman's respect for the children's abilities grew with her experience as their teacher. The second annual report included her comments on the importance of good teachers for the children:

> The right spirit and the energy are all there, if only the ideal teacher could be found to develop them. Such a teacher would be wise enough and patient enough to discover the needs of the individual child, and meet them. She would be sympathetic enough to enter into play as she does into study, to be ready to throw herself into

anything from multiplication tables to digging a garden. Above all, sensible enough not to regard the children hysterically as "unfortunate wretches," but keeping in her own mind their limitations, try to prevent in them any morbid reflections, and in all things to deal with them as sanely and lovingly as though they were her own.[16]

The long stays at the hospital began to tax the facilities of City and County Hospital. The initial ward for Gillette's patients was followed within two years by the construction of an open-air screened pavilion, and then the exclusive use of a small, separate building on the grounds. In each annual report, Dr. Gillette and the regents acknowledged without reservation the support that had been provided by Dr. Ancker and his staff at City and County

> *The school department of the State Hospital for Crippled Children is surely past the experimental stage, having completed nearly the fourth year of its existence. It has established itself as an important adjunct to medical treatment, besides giving to such children as are able to receive it the beginning of the education that is their right.*
>
> **Frances Boardman, Teacher**
> **6th Annual Report, 1903**

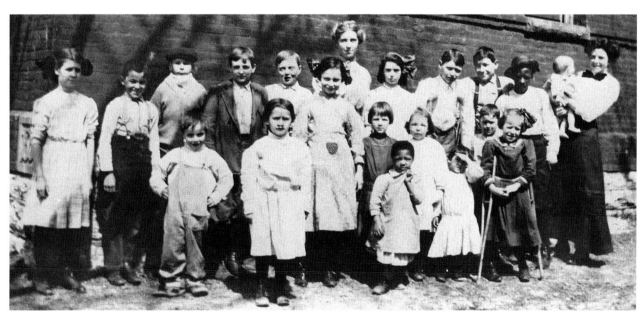

Class and teachers, circa 1900

Hospital, but despite this a series of events were unfolding which would end with a move to a new site.[17]

In 1905 the legislature noted the growth of the State Hospital for Crippled and Deformed Children and on March 25 appointed a legislative commission of three members to "investigate and report upon the advisability of establishing a state hospital for crippled, indigent, and deformed children in Ramsey County." The three commissioners were Arthur Gillette, Stephen Mahoney, and Dr. Robert Earl, a surgeon who practiced in St. Paul and a friend of Gillette. The implications of the charge to the commission must have created second thoughts, for on April 5 a second act was passed which expanded the scope of the search to include Hennepin County. The commission was told to report its conclusions during the 1907 legislative session.[18]

The move to include Hennepin County in the search for a new site may have come from the University of Minnesota. In 1905 the university received a gift of $112,000 from the estate of Dr. A. F. Elliot for the purpose of building a memorial hospital on university grounds. The regents were uncertain of their authority to receive and administer such a designated gift. In 1901 a bill was introduced in the legislature to create a single State Board of Control to manage the state's charitable institutions. While most of these institutions had been well managed, the endless appeals for funding from each of the institutional governing boards had frustrated legislators. Their frustration extended to the University of Minnesota, and the original bill was amended to place the university, all normal schools, and the state soldiers' home under the

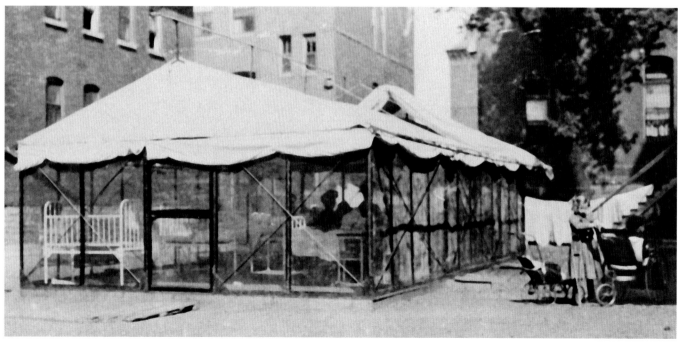

Open-air pavilion, circa 1900

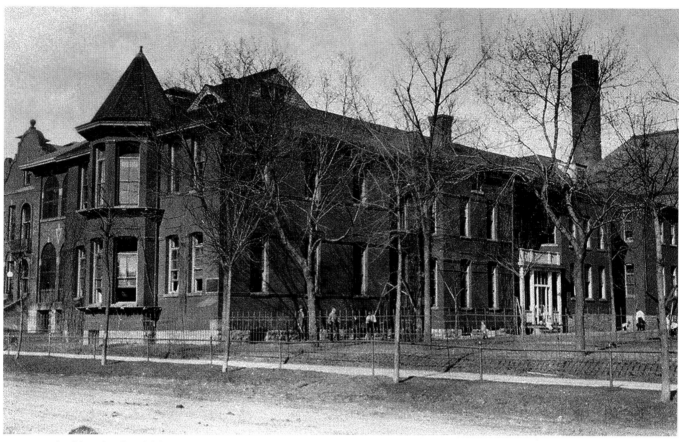

Two-story building for the children, 1911

financial supervision of the State Board of Control. The result was that the regents retained authority in educational matters, but the State Board of Control managed the university budget and reviewed every funding request. A bitter fight followed, and in 1905 the Board of Control was relieved of its financial supervision of the university. The regents then asked the legislature to accept the Elliot bequest and turn the funds over to the university to determine what sort of hospital should be built.[19]

Within the University's College of Medicine and Surgery the faculty was excited by the prospect of a hospital at the university. There was debate about its location and size and the allocation of beds for medical and surgical care. It must have seemed logical to the faculty that the legislative commission would seriously consider the Elliot Memorial Hospital as the site for a new hospital for crippled and deformed children. After all, the commission included a regent in Stephen Mahoney and a member of the medical faculty executive committee in Arthur Gillette. Dr. Gillette must have received considerable pressure, for at the faculty executive committee meeting on December 7, 1906, he felt obliged to announce that he intended to write to each faculty member and explain his position on the matter. That correspondence has been lost. The regents made their position clear in a meeting on February 20, 1907. They passed a resolution offering the legislative commission land adjacent to the site of the proposed Elliot Memorial Hospital, and "urged and recommended that said Hospital for Crippled and Deformed Children be located on said site." To make it more attractive to Dr. Gillette, they offered to retain the retiring Stephen Mahoney as a liaison between the board of regents and the crippled children's hospital.[20]

However, City and County Hospital did not want to lose the hospital for crippled children, and in 1906 the Ramsey County Board of Control erected a two-story brick building to accommodate its growth and provide classroom space. By that time, more than 350 children had received care and there were 65 children in the hospital. The new building even included an x-ray unit, a very new technology at that time, and the annual report for 1906 cited fifty-six radiographs that had been performed to assess deformities. On March 7, 1907, the city of St. Paul offered the legislative commission the brick buildings currently occupied by the hospital and 4.5 acres of adjacent land at City and County Hospital for future expansion. Dr. Ancker also agreed to continue the 1897 weekly patient charges for an additional five years.[21]

It is likely that Dr. Gillette did not favor a move to the new hospital at the university simply because it didn't fit his vision of the future. His annual reports as surgeon-in-chief had called attention to the problem of preparing the children to support themselves after their medical care was complete. In the annual report of 1907, he became more vocal in his concern:

> The other states which have followed our [medical] example have rather surpassed us in one respect. . . . There are many individual cases in mind of children who are at present helpless cripples, who are helpless not only physically but financially, for whom the state has made no provision whatever. An industrial school for cripples would educate these as they are educated and cared for in England, Ireland, Philadelphia, and Massachusetts. We could teach them typewriting, typesetting, basket making, carpet and rug weaving, dress making, plain sewing, shoe making and all kinds of leather work, tailoring, clay modeling, and for the girls dress making, millinery, cooking, baking, housekeeping, etc. For those tuberculously inclined we could teach farming, gardening, floriculture, care of poultry and dairying.

Gillette envisioned a staged process of rehabilitation, with medical care followed by the acquisition of practical job skills. In his mind, those skills were best taught in a fresh air parkland environment separate from a hospital. The offer of the city of St. Paul and City and County Hospital also did not fulfill Gillette's ideal, although they were familiar partners. He knew that the university

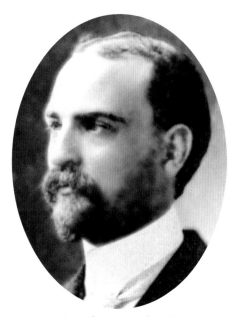

Dr. Robert O. Earl, 1902

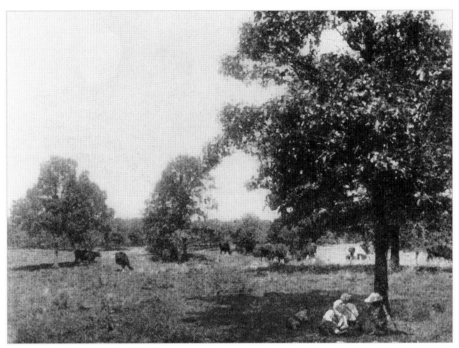

The twenty-three acres at Phalen Park, 1909 (see Appendix D)

had no experience in running a hospital, and that there was no room for vocational training in the Elliot hospital.[22]

The St. Paul community was Gillette's best hope for making his industrial school a reality. St. Paul was the place where he lived and worked, and where he had strong social connections with organizations such as the Commercial Club and the Business League. Dr. Robert Earl, the third member of the legislative commission, may have been sympathetic to Gillette's desire to keep the hospital and school in St. Paul. In the future, Earl would provide surgical care for the children as a member of the hospital's medical staff. As a member of the St. Paul Parks Commission, he was familiar with sites that could satisfy Gillette's vision. One in particular was Phalen Park, at that time on the edge of the city. The city of

St. Paul, anticipating growth in that direction, was creating a large park on the western shore of Lake Phalen, with most of the land acquired through condemnation proceedings. One owner who was forced to give up land was Reuben Warner, a well-known St. Paul businessman who lost seventeen acres to park development in 1900. Warner died in 1901, and in his estate his residual property adjacent to the park went to his children. One of Warner's relatives, Eli Warner, was an officer of the Commercial Club in 1907 when the club, the Business League, and "certain citizens" offered the legislative commission up to five thousand dollars to acquire the twenty-three acres held by the Reuben Warner estate and build a fresh air sanitarium or cottage.[23]

On April 2, 1907, the legislature passed a bill accepting a joint offer from the city of St. Paul,

If you think $15,000 a year will carry us through, do not make it any more, for I believe we do not, this year, want to make it any larger than we can help. Pardon this suggestion.

**Dr. Arthur Gillette
to Stephen Mahoney, 1907**

I wish also to state that you did a great act of kindness when you admitted this child into the State Hospital temporarily. Even though the father is able to care for the child financially, there are times, and such was the condition when I last saw this man, when he is not mentally competent due to a fluid frequently taken by individuals to stimulate their oversensitive natures.

**Dr. Arthur Gillette
to State Board of Control, 1912**

City and County Hospital, the Commercial Club, and the Business League. In a series of transactions on June 3 and 4, the heirs of Reuben Warner transferred their land parcels to the state at a total cost of $4,725.[24] By December 1907 the Commercial Club and Business League had raised the funds to meet their commitment to the state to reimburse the cost of this purchase. The city of St. Paul was to provide the state with land for a new building, but was slow to take action and did not complete its transfer of the deeds to City and County Hospital property until August 4, 1908. The 1907 legislative action also changed the name of the hospital to the State Hospital for Indigent Crippled and Deformed Children.[25] But the biggest surprise was a change in governance. Perhaps responding to the board of regents' long-standing request to be freed of the responsibility of supervising a crippled children's hospital, or perhaps anticipating that the regents would have enough to do supervising the Elliot Memorial Hospital, the legislature assigned the governance of the hospital for crippled children to the State Board of Control. Arthur Gillette's easy and effective working relationship with Stephen Mahoney ended.[26]

The State Board of Control began to exercise its authority immediately. A meeting on May 27, 1907, resulted in restructuring the hospital administration. In addition to the surgeon-in-chief position, a superintendent posi-

tion was created and given to Arthur Ancker. The superintendent held significant power, and the position was a direct challenge to Dr. Gillette's authority. As described in the minutes of the meeting, "the superintendent . . . shall be its chief executive officer, and under the direction of the State Board of Control shall have general supervision and control of all the departments of the said hospital, of all officers, employees and patients, and charge of the grounds, buildings and equipment thereof." In addition, "the superintendent of the hospital shall be the authorized means of communication between the State Board of Control . . . in all matters relating to the welfare of the hospital." By comparison, "the surgeon-in-chief [is] to have general charge and supervision of the medical and surgical treatment of patients admitted to such hospital."[27]

Ancker probably enjoyed his new role. His 1908 annual report to the State Board of Control opened with a letter in which he asked the board to immediately take action to construct a new hospital building on the property at City and County Hospital that had been given to the state for that purpose. Gillette's report was devoted exclusively to the need for an industrial school and made no mention of hospital conditions at City and County Hospital. Both doctors expressed appreciation for each other in generous words that gave no hint of any conflict between them. That may have reflected the public civility

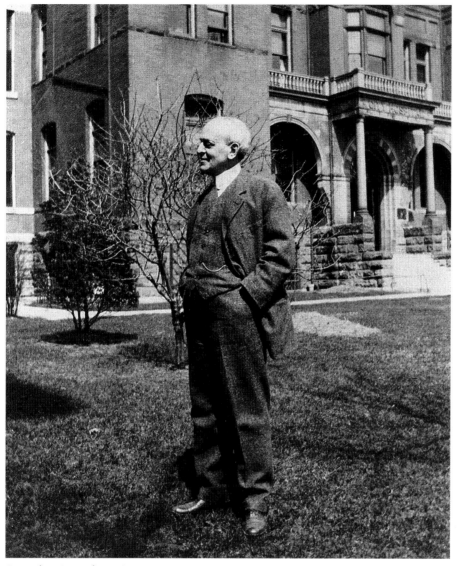

Dr. Arthur B. Ancker, 1911

Board of Control, which he did. He said they got out to the meeting and Dr. Ancker said "I'd like to take you gentlemen over to the Minnesota State Hospital for Crippled Children and see how these children are faring." He said they went over and the children had their plates filled with turkey, potatoes and five times as much as they could eat for any dinner, just heaped up in grand style. Then he went back to the meeting, and Dr. Ancker, in front of the Board of Control, stated: "This young surgeon has the audacity to complain about the type of food that I'm feeding these children!" Dr. Gillette said that he was so mad that he went right down to the Commercial Club and secured his funds, and the Commercial Club also got it arranged so that 23 acres of land which was a frog pond was donated to the State of Minnesota for the building of a new hospital.[29]

and graciousness of the times, for conflict was present.[28]

More than fifty years later, Dr. Carl Chatterton, Dr. Gillette's successor as surgeon-in-chief, remembered an event which may have been the breaking point in the relationship between Ancker and Gillette:

Dr. Gillette told me the reason the children were finally moved out to Phalen Park was because of the fact that

he went out to the Minnesota State Hospital For Crippled Children, then located at the City and County Hospital grounds one afternoon and found that the children, for dinner, were having a slice of bread without any butter or milk, and that was all. He complained bitterly to Dr. Ancker and about two weeks later Dr. Gillette got an invitation to come out to Ancker Hospital to meet the

It is impossible to verify this story, but no money was ever appropriated to build a new hospital at City and County Hospital. In 1909 the legislature did appropriate fifty-five thousand dollars for a "fresh air sanitarium and educational and industrial school building for the indigent crippled and deformed children of the State of Minnesota." This building was placed on the property near Lake Phalen which had been purchased from the Warner estate.[30] In his annual report for 1910, Dr. Ancker described the structures used by the children at City and County as "entirely inadequate." In an effort to pressure the state to build a new children's hospital on the City and County Hospital site, in addition to the school and sanitarium at Lake Phalen, the Ramsey County Board of Control threatened to not renew its contract with the state to provide care in the buildings occupied at City and County Hospital. The contract was due to expire on January 1, 1913, and as a commissioner put it: "I am not going to be a party to running a firetrap for these children a day longer than is necessary." A joint meeting of the two boards failed to result in a commitment from the state to build at City and County Hospital. The city of St. Paul took legal action to reclaim the donated land and buildings at City and County Hospital, and the legislature agreed to return them.[31]

The hospital's 1912 annual report is conspicuous for the absence of any report from Dr. Ancker. Dr. Gillette attempted to put a positive spin on the situation:

As the Ramsey County Board of Control does not wish to renew its contract for board and care of the children, and as a bill was introduced in the last legislature asking that the hospital of one hundred beds on the grounds of City and County Hospital be returned to Ramsey County, which bill was passed by the legislature, we will be left January 1, 1913, without sufficient room to care for our patients . . . but there was also donated money toward the building of a hospital and school [at Phalen Park], which is now fully equipped, and is caring for a large number of children. We now require on these grounds extra wards. We can use the same building for cooking and dining rooms, and also use one heating plant. . . . In short, to double the work we are now doing for the indigent crippled and deformed children of Minnesota we ask only four small wards of twenty-five beds each, adjoining the present main building, with an extra story on the present executive building for the nurses and help.[32]

By 1914 the transition was complete. Gillette and Ancker saw the results differently. In his 1914 annual report to the State Board of Control, Dr. Gillette stated: "The State of Minnesota has reason to be proud of the 160 bed Hospital now erected at Phalen Park, and almost complete." In his annual report to the Ramsey County Board of Control, Dr. Ancker stated: "In this report are included that of the City and County Hospital in all its departments, the Hospital for the Crippled and Deformed Children having been abandoned by the State, so far as this hospital is concerned, and transferred to its new home at Lake Phalen in the month of December, last."

For the first time in twenty years Arthur Gillette was not listed in the 1914 City and County Hospital Annual Report as the hospital orthopaedic surgeon. His name was replaced by those of Carl Chatterton and Wallace Cole.

The Order of Things

As the city of St. Paul prospered, there was a need for new homes for its residents and new buildings for its businesses. Many of these buildings were designed by the prolific and versatile St. Paul architect Clarence Johnston. Although less well-known than his friend Cass Gilbert, who designed the current Minnesota State Capitol, Johnston served as state architect from 1901 through 1931.

In his career Johnston designed and supervised construction of buildings at virtually every facility managed by the State Board of Control. Nearly all the buildings at the Phalen site of the crippled children's hospital, as well as many of the buildings at the hospital's first home, City and County Hospital, were designed by Johnston. According to Paul Clifford Larson, author of *Minnesota Architect: The Life and Work of Clarence H. Johnston*, the architect began his state projects by considering the purpose of the building. He preferred solid construction that did not require complicated maintenance.

The buildings also were designed to accommodate changes in institutional needs. Appearance was a lower, but important, priority.[1] A characteristic of Johnston's work for the State Board of Control was the completion of projects under budget. The 1909 legislature appropriated $55,000 for the initial Phalen construction. The first buildings at Phalen were designed by Johnston in 1910 and constructed at a cost of $48,265. The move from the City and County Hospital site required changes in these first buildings. Portions of them were remodeled and new buildings were added.

This was completed by 1915 at a cost of $58,000, and allowed the hospitalization of an additional one hundred children, since the space at City and County Hospital had limited the number of children who could receive care there.[2] The new facility at Lake Phalen had much more room, which resulted in a rapid increase in the number of admissions. During 1917 and 1918, 426 children were admitted, including 358 who were admitted for the first time. On a typical day there were 138 children in the hospital, and they stayed an average of 260 days. The most common reason for admission was tuberculosis, often referred to as consumption.[3]

Tuberculosis, with its fever, cough, blood-spitting, weight loss, and draining skin lesions from bone infection, had been known for a long time but was not widespread until the late 1800s. The tuberculosis epidemic followed the changes in society brought about by the Industrial Revolution. Those most at risk were the poor, the malnourished, and those living and working in crowded, poorly ventilated, and unsanitary conditions. The cause, a rod-shaped bacterium called Mycobacterium tuberculosis, had been discovered by the German physician Robert Koch and report-

ed in 1882, but the discovery was not followed by a remedy. Numerous quack cures were sold by both charlatans and well-trained physicians, but an effective medicine, streptomycin, would not be found until the 1940s. Instead, treatment focused on a healthy lifestyle, an effort that reached its pinnacle in the tuberculosis sanitarium, a place where every detail of daily life was organized around the goal of getting well.[4]

The mandate of the Hospital for Indigent Crippled and Deformed Children to serve the poorest children of Minnesota brought large numbers of youngsters with tuberculosis to the hospital. Between 1897 and 1928, a total

of 892 children with tuberculosis received care. Tuberculosis admissions increased steadily from 1897 to a peak of fifty-four admissions in 1919, steadily decreased until the 1940s, and nearly disappeared after antibiotics became available. Children with active tuberculosis of the lung were not accepted, but those children with tuberculosis of the bones were not considered infectious, and were placed on the wards with other children. Tuberculosis most often invaded the spine, or the ends of the long bones of the arms and legs. Spinal tuberculosis, or Pott's disease, destroyed the vertebrae and allowed the spine to collapse into sharply angulated deformities,

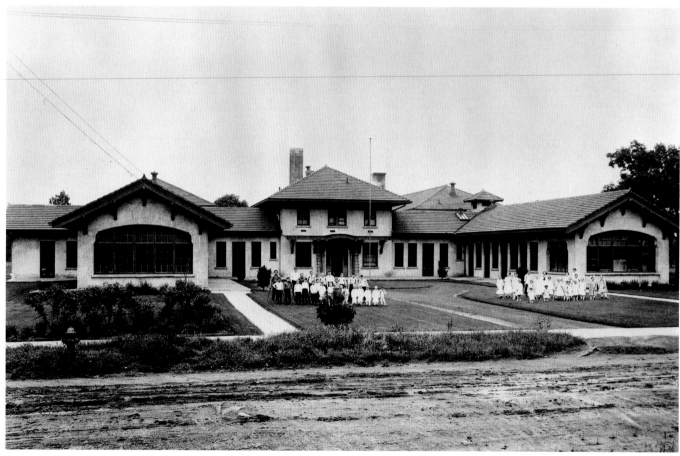

State Hospital for Indigent Crippled and Deformed Children, 1916

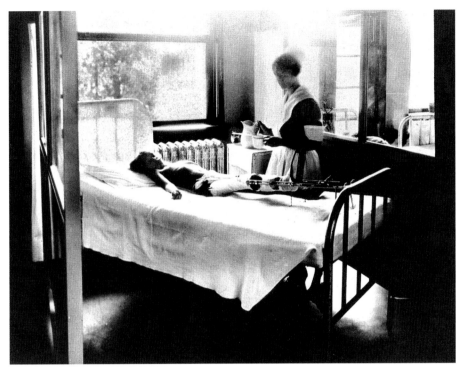
A young boy in traction, circa 1920

often paralyzing the legs. Tuberculosis of the long bones destroyed joints, resulting in stiff or contracted arms and legs that made everyday activities like walking impossible. The bony abscesses of tuberculosis frequently worked their way to the skin and drained through sores that would not heal.[5]

Tuberculosis was not the only problem seen at the hospital. Children were admitted with other types of bone infection, referred to as osteomyelitis. They received care for clubfoot, dislocation of the hip, deformities after fractures, bad scars after burns, cleft lip and palate, scoliosis or curvature of the spine, paralysis due to poliomyelitis, and deformities due to the spasticity of cerebral palsy. Occasionally a child was admitted with cancer of the bone, and the hospital then became a hospice, a place of gentle care until death.[6]

The State Board of Control met with its superintendents and officers every three months at one of the state institutions. The meetings were recorded by a stenographer, and the minutes published, much like courtroom proceedings. The meeting of November 2, 1915, was held at Phalen Park and offers a priceless insight into the work of the hospital. Dr. Gillette was asked to conduct a tour and describe the children's problems. He began with a plea: "There are one or two things I wish to speak about in here. The first is that these children do not suffer. Do not look upon them as little sufferers and weep. We have people who do that. They will look at the children and say: 'You poor little sufferers!' The children cannot understand what they are talking about." He then took them through the wards, describing each child from memory and lingering on children who were special successes: "This boy has a tuberculous disease of the cervical vertebrae. He is wearing this brace because we want to keep his head on top of his shoulders. There was complete paralysis at one time. Can you wiggle

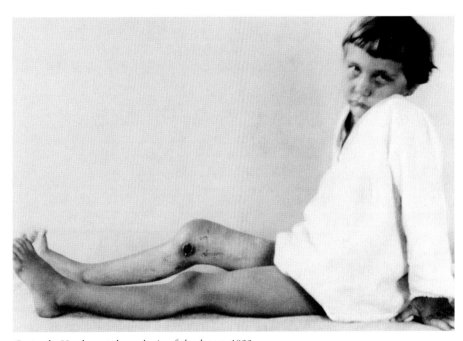
Gertrude Honken, tuberculosis of the knee, 1923

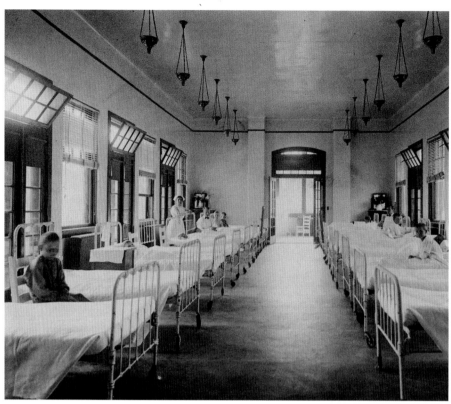

A boys ward, 1915

your toes, boy? That little motion is worth about $20,000 to the state. We expect that boy to get well." A girl with weakness from polio also received special mention. Through surgery the tendons of the strong muscles in her forearm were redirected to give her useful strength in her hands, which Dr. Gillette promptly demonstrated. He also acknowledged the work of others. The first child ever to undergo spine fusion surgery at the hospital was present, and he credited Dr. Chatterton with performing the surgery.

The emphasis on providing care to children who could benefit and become more self-sufficient was evident. The tour group encountered a child with cerebral palsy, and Dr. Gillette took the opportunity to make a statement.

"I want to talk to you a little regarding these cases of cerebral palsy. We are constantly getting applications to admit these children. When the parents write us that they have a child that cannot walk and cannot talk and wish to have the child admitted to this institution, I write back and ask if the child is bright. You know what they always say: 'It is the brightest child in the family.' And when you see the child you pity the rest." Gillette's comment was insensitive, but it was typical of the strong bias against the mentally impaired that was held by most people at that time. Children who were considered "spastic" or "retarded" were often kept at home or sent to state institutions where they lived out of sight of society.

Dr. Gillette, who knew his audience, took the opportunity to demonstrate his concern for expenses. Because the move to Phalen meant that surgery had to be performed at the new site, the tour group inspected the new operating room. Dr. Gillette described its creation: "This is the operating room, which of course, you recognize at once. I got a man who had charge of an operating room to come see what he could do for us. He told us he could fix up an operating room, which he thought would be satisfactory, for eleven thousand dollars. Well, I have a good deal of nerve, but I did not have nerve enough to tell the board of control that we wanted eleven thousand dollars for an operating room. The board allowed me plenty of money, but not eleven thousand dollars for an operating room, and we fitted up this room for much less, and we do all the kinds of

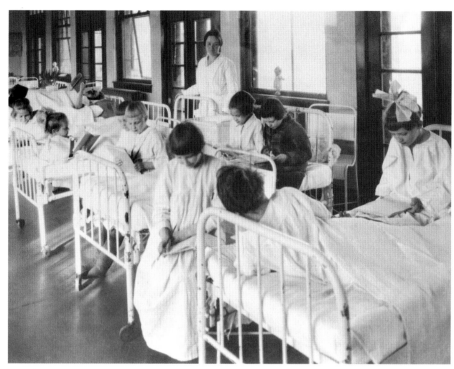

A girls ward, circa 1920

operating that we wish."

A visit to the brace department drove Dr. Gillette's point home: "This is the instrument department, a room for making appliances and where we manu-

facture all of our braces now. We have only one man in charge, and he does not come every day. We find that older boys are a great help to him, and the girls do a great deal of sewing. In that way we save a great deal of money, besides keeping the patients more or less busy."[7]

The life of the hospital at Lake Phalen had become much more complicated than at City and County Hospital. Before the need to move from City and County was clear, the Phalen site was to have been an industrial school. With the transfer of all activity to Phalen, the focus had changed. The Phalen site would have to be more than a temporary home for children who had recovered from an illness and were receiving job skills before returning home. The buildings at Phalen became a hospital, with nurses, therapists,

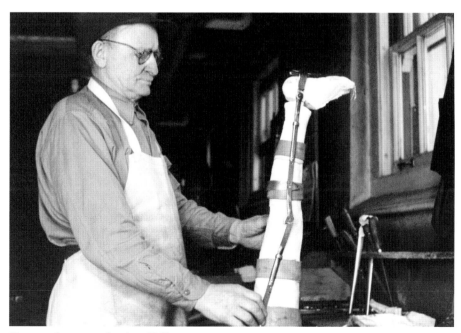

Brace maker at work, circa 1940

cooks, maids, secretaries, grounds keepers, and maintenance men. The new campus needed an administrator, someone with a firm hand to take charge of the changes and supervise the growth of the hospital. Dr. Gillette found just such a person in Elizabeth McGregor.

Born in St. Cloud, Minnesota, on August 19, 1875, Elizabeth McGregor was the oldest of seven children. Her parents later moved to a homestead near Hawley, Minnesota. Her mother died in 1891, and, according to their grandniece Donna Christianson, Elizabeth and her sister Margaret assumed responsibility for the younger children in the family when they disapproved of their father's plan to remarry. Elizabeth worked as a teacher in neighboring rural school districts, and then attended the University of

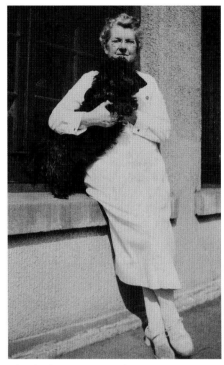

Elizabeth McGregor, administrator, 1938

Minnesota, where her course work included economics, ethics, sociology, finance, and psychology. She graduated in 1901 with a bachelor's degree in philosophy. From 1901 to 1908 Elizabeth taught in elementary schools on the west side of St. Paul and attended graduate courses in social work at the University of Minnesota. In 1908 she took a position at the State School for Dependent and Neglected Children at Owatonna. She served as superintendent there from 1911 to 1914.[8]

It is likely that Elizabeth knew of the changes at the Phalen campus through her work at Owatonna. The State Board of Control's regular meetings with the superintendents of the state facilities may have provided her with an opportunity to meet Dr. Gillette. In 1914 she was recruited to become superintendent of the hospital at Phalen Park. She refused the job, then

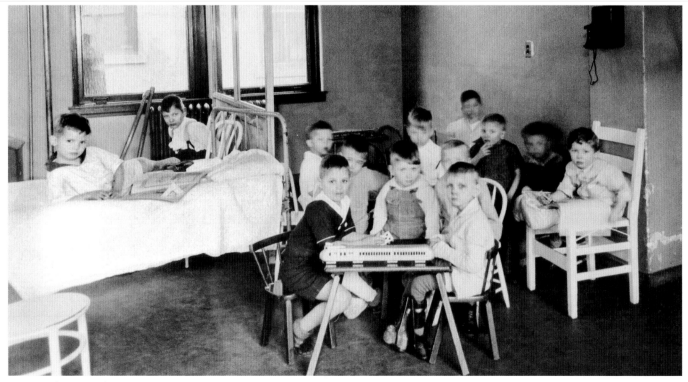

Younger boys ward, 1937

reconsidered, accepted the post, and was sent by Dr. Gillette on a four-month tour of Europe to study hospital management. Elizabeth returned to St. Paul on September 29, 1914, and started work the next day. She must have been desperately needed. In a 1944 newspaper article, Elizabeth was quoted as saying, "If I'd had fifteen minutes free time to get downtown any day during the first three months I spent here, they'd never have seen me again."[9]

Miss McGregor, as she would be known to everyone at the hospital for the next thirty-five years, was the perfect choice. She had no medical experience, and that allowed Dr. Gillette to assume responsibility for medical decisions. She was a skillful administrator and a hard worker who had unchallenged authority over the daily affairs of the hospital. The 1916 biennial report demonstrated the demands of her job and her attention to detail. Her superintendent's report covered everything,

including the grounds and buildings, educational work, religious instruction for the children, and recreation. It also carefully outlined the needs of the hospital. She requested a new school building, the original facility having been turned over to hospital care, and a greenhouse to grow vegetables during the winter and flowers for the wards. She asked for funds to establish a program to visit the home of every child admitted to the hospital. She recognized that the work done at the hospital would be lost if a child went home to a poor environment.

The grounds and buildings were a constant concern. The pressure to admit more children grew every year, requiring the construction of a west wing in 1920-21 at a cost of $91,000, and an east wing in 1924-25 at a cost of $96,000. By 1926 there were 233 children in the hospital on an average day. Support service buildings were needed, including a powerhouse ($39,000 in 1918), a

Won't you please make a plea to have that word "indigent" struck out? It is an ugly word at best.

**Mrs. George Welch
Superintendent, Fergus Falls
State Hospital, 1915**

If we attempt to change the word "indigent," what better word can we find to express the thought? Its synonyms are needy, poverty stricken, destitute, etc. We will run up against difficulties if we try to change our nomenclature. The only way to remove the words that are so objectionable is to remove the poverty and social conditions which make them necessary.

**Reverend A. J. D. Haupt
1915**

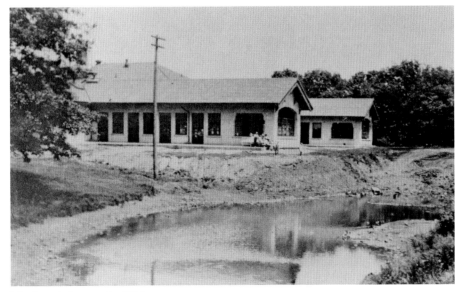

The hospital grounds, 1913

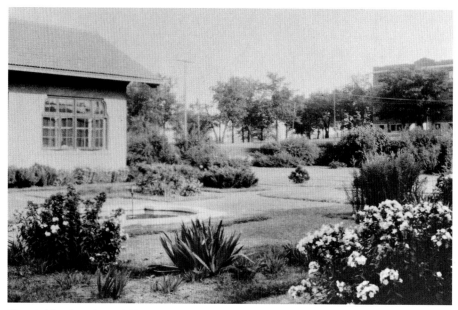

Hospital landscaping, 1925

general service building ($81,000 in 1921), and a laundry ($21,000 in 1923). She found it necessary to look after every detail of the campus. Rats and mice were a constant nuisance around the garbage areas, and the root cellar never seemed to keep the fruits and vegetables at just the right temperature. Ivy Avenue, in front of the hospital, wasn't paved and often was in poor condition. In a letter to the board of control, Miss McGregor pointed out that "There are times when delivery is difficult and during the wet season, almost impossible. We have had heavy trucks drive down the sidewalk on account of the difficulty of getting through the mud in the street."

At heart Miss McGregor was a gardener. When a greenhouse was constructed in 1918, she constantly looked for opportunities to beautify the grounds. Trees were planted, and low spots on the grounds were filled in with dirt excavated from public projects around the city. She solicited advice from professional landscape workers, and received advice from Eloise Butler about a wildflower garden. She planted strawberries, gooseberries, blackberries, raspberries, currants, and rhubarb by the hundreds. She convinced the St. Paul parks commission to plant a border of Siberian pea trees, white and pink lilacs, spirea, and buckthorn along the fence behind the hospital property. She asked experts at the University of Minnesota's St. Paul campus to describe the qualifications of a professional gardener, then appealed to the board of control to employ a man at a salary of one hundred dollars a month. The hospital dentist, working half time, was paid fifty dollars a month.

The neighboring park and golf course were very troublesome. Park visitors walked across the lawn and scattered debris on the grounds. Popcorn vendors stationed themselves just down the street, and on Sundays beggars sat at the end of the driveway where visitors entered. Miss McGregor complained bitterly to the board of control: "We take care of the grounds from the inside to the best of our ability with the help we have. . . . Bottles, partly eaten lunches, papers, empty boxes etc. are thrown into our hedge, over our fence, and on our boulevard by the passers-by on their way to and from the park. I have taken this matter up with the park authorities many times." The golf course caddies were just as bad. Miss McGregor wrote to the parks commissioner: "We are very much annoyed by the boys who serve as caddies on the Golf Links. They cut through our hedge and peony beds for a short cut to the park. We strongly object to having any-one cut across our grounds and ask your cooperation in trying to put a stop to it."

High quality food for the children was a major concern. The hospital gardens covered nine

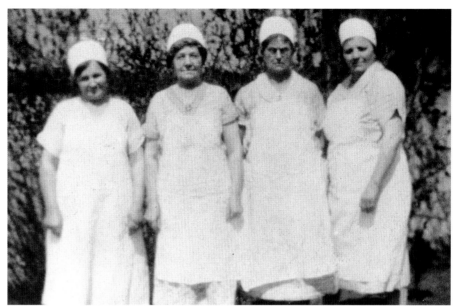

The cooks, 1938

acres at their largest, and supplied vegetables for the kitchen. Meat, flour, milk, and other foods were bought from suppliers through the State Board of Control, but deliveries often were unpredictable, and the quality of the food was uneven. As an example, surplus canned bacon from the War Department was fatty and was rejected. Milk was particularly important, and

Miss McGregor could not find a suitable vendor until the milk was purchased bottled and pasteurized. The board of control was worried about the cost, but Miss McGregor had bulk milk samples tested and could document contamination that alarmed the doctors. Flour purchased in bulk was also of inconsistent quality, and bread often became moldy. Miss

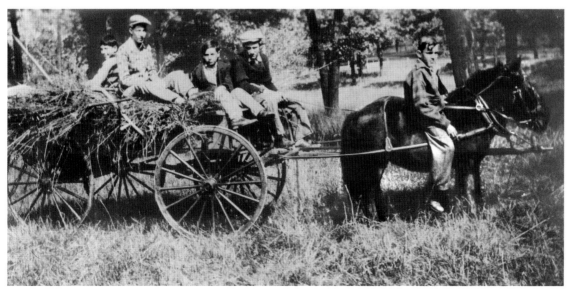

Boys at work in the yard, 1938

McGregor sent samples to the University of Minnesota and to Dunwoody Institute. She corresponded extensively with the board of control and the Pillsbury Flour Mill Company until she received flour of the quality she desired. The Kellogg Toasted Corn Flake Company sent her a case of products to taste in hopes that purchases would follow, but she was above being bribed. She found them "all excellent," but didn't order them.

By 1923 the hospital had 115 employees, and Miss McGregor was responsible for each one. Each had a job description, but most found themselves helping out in other areas, too. As many as thirty or forty of the employees lived at the hospital and received room and board as a part of their compensation. Work days were long, with shifts often lasting ten or twelve hours. Salaries as state employees were never high, and Miss McGregor often found herself explaining to the board of control why raises were deserved. In 1924 custodians were paid $40 per month, stenographers and librarians $50 per month, laundry workers $54 per month, porters $73 per month, assistant engineers $82 per month, the chief engineer $120 per month, and the supervisor of nurses $135 per month. Miss McGregor herself was paid $200 a month. Hard work and loyalty were valued. Many appeals to the board of control cited the length of service and work ethic of an employee.

On the other hand, Elizabeth McGregor wasn't shy about pointing out deficiencies in an employee's performance. In 1915 the hospital created a brace shop, and the surgeon-in-chief hired a brace maker to reduce the cost of braces built by private firms in St. Paul. The department created 332 braces and appliances in 1917 and 1918 and 1,112 braces and appliances in 1919 and 1920. Since outpatient clinics were held on Thursdays, families and medical staff began to complain about the time it took for a brace to be built or repaired. In 1921 George Allard, the brace maker, described his problems in a letter to Miss McGregor: "The hospital patient and outpatient departments are requiring too many braces for me to make

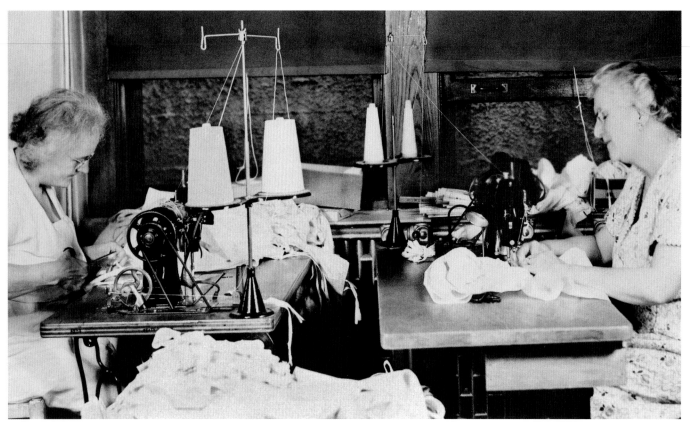

Ladies sewing, circa 1940

promptly. I think the best way to do would be to hire some extra help. I can get a competent man to work extra time 15 hours per week at 65 cents per hour. Some weeks I would not need him as many hours . . . I would also recommend some different arrangements be made for handling the Thursday afternoon repair work. It is almost impossible to do all the repair work in a few hours."

Miss McGregor promised to take the matter up with the State Board of Control. She analyzed Allard's work volume and told the board not to grant more money for brace work. Her response to Allard was quite blunt: "I am in receipt of advice from the board of control concerning extra help in your department. Inasmuch as the work has been materially lighter during the past three months, no extra help or increase in salary paid in this department will be allowed. However, we expect loyalty, and prompt and efficient service. Outpatients cannot be held over for two or three days or a week for repairs or adjustments that require only a short time to make." The problems of the brace department continued for many years.

In 1922 Miss McGregor opened the hospital to inspection by the American College of Surgeons, which, in an effort to improve the care in American hospitals, inspected hospitals and issued certificates of quality. The State Hospital for Indigent Crippled and Deformed Children was given a Class A certificate, the highest possible ranking. Even so, the

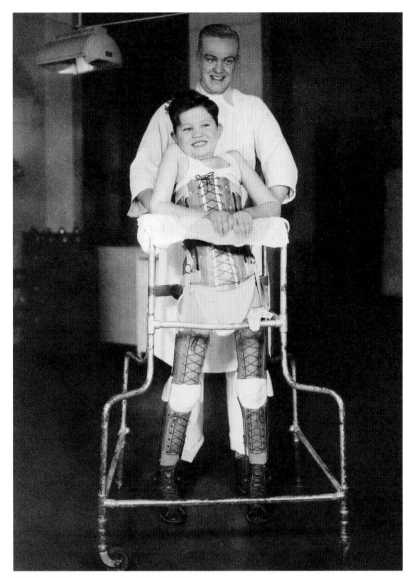

Child with braces and walker, 1940

board of control occasionally received complaints, most of them about messy wards, nursing care, the quality of the food, or visiting hours. These were routinely referred to Miss McGregor, who responded to each one in detail. Some of the concerns were valid. The number of patients had steadily increased so that by 1926 there were 233 children in the hospital each day. The care they required had become very complicated. On a typical day a child required

more than being fed, bathed, and clothed. Dressings were changed, braces applied, casts inspected. Therapy sessions were balanced against schoolwork. Staff doctors appeared on the ward at any time, and Miss McGregor insisted that a nurse accompany the doctor during rounds. The doctors dictated all their orders, which were then written or typed in the chart.

Miss McGregor found it difficult to recruit competent and diligent nurses and maids for the

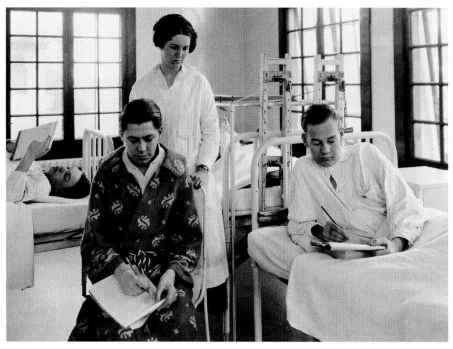

Patients and high school teacher, 1921

At the heart of Miss McGregor's struggle with the nursing staff was her desire to increase the competence of the average nurse. Bothered by the poor training of the nurses she hired, she came to assume that the average nurse knew nothing about the special problems of the children in the hospital. Her background as a teacher emerged in her plan to create a nursing school, a sort of post-graduate or finishing school for nurses where they might sharpen their skills before seeking a job. The course of study varied from two months to six months, and the curriculum was intense. Lectures were given in pediatric and orthopaedic medicine, bibliotherapy, oral hygiene, dietetics, and occupational and physical therapy. The nursing school was approved by the State Board of Control in 1921, and Miss McGregor placed responsibility for the school in the

wards, and the nursing staff struggled under her firm hand and scrutiny of detail. Marie Hoppe was the first matron or supervising nurse in the Phalen building. She stayed on in the capacity of superintendent of nurses after the hospital work was transferred from City and County Hospital to the newly expanded Phalen complex. She had a good relationship with Miss McGregor, and she served as the hospital's acting superintendent when Miss McGregor was in military service in 1918. As a Red Cross volunteer, Miss McGregor was assigned to organize aid for displaced women and children near the battle lines in France. Marie Hoppe took on new responsibilities after her return, including administering anesthesia during surgery, performing x-rays, and supervising the drug room.

Miss McGregor took personal responsibility for the nurses, but she found the extra responsibility a burden, and hired a new superintendent of nurses. In the span of three years, at least five nursing superintendents came and went, and at least two nursing superintendents wrote to the State Board of Control to explain their resignation. Celestine Keefe was the most descriptive: "I cannot continue my duties as Superintendent of Nurses. . . . Practically speaking, there seems to be no particular need of a Superintendent of Nurses as the work ordinarily in that department is entirely taken care of by the business Superintendent . . . my spirit was generally killed, and my initiative was needless, as well as killed. As a result the atmosphere has become most unpleasant, resulting I should say from my not simply accepting all orders and very severe reprimands, which one ordinarily would not hear given to a grown-up, let alone one who is presumably a lady."

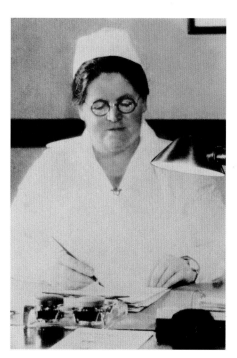

Margaret McGregor, 1930

hands of the superintendent of nurses. This made that job impossible. Caring for the daily nursing needs of the children was a big job, and teaching graduate nurses was work that a natural educator like Miss McGregor would scrutinize closely. No average human being could succeed in the job of superintendent of nurses. So, in October 1922 Elizabeth turned to her sister Margaret to take on the job.[10]

Margaret McGregor graduated from the nursing school at St. Luke's Hospital in St. Paul in 1905. For many years she worked as a private duty nurse in hospitals in Minneapolis and St. Paul. Margaret became a Red Cross volunteer in 1917 and preceded Elizabeth to France, where she served the wounded. After the war she studied public health nursing at the University of Minnesota, and then worked briefly as a public health nurse in Kalispell, Montana. In 1921 she rejoined the Red Cross and was sent to Estonia, where she organized nursing services during war restoration efforts. When she returned to St. Paul in September 1922, she had no firm plans and was willing to listen to Elizabeth's request for help. Beyond being Elizabeth's sister, Margaret's nursing experience and organizational skills made her a good choice for the job of superintendent of nurses. Her appointment brought relative peace to the nursing staff and the nursing school for the next twenty years.[11]

During the 1920s the hospital was open to visitors daily from 9 a. m. to 9 p. m., with the exception of Thursday morning, which was reserved for rounds of the wards by the staff doctors. Wednesday and Sunday visiting hours were restricted to parents, but for many children there were few family visits. Long distance travel was difficult, and some children didn't see their parents from the day of admission to the day of discharge. When families did visit, brothers and sisters were not allowed in. This irritated many parents and other adults. On one occasion, a physician wrote a letter to the editor of the *Saint Paul Dispatch* to complain about the policy. Under the headline "Sisters Kept Apart: Doctor Writes That State Hospital for Crippled Children Has Cruel Rules," Dr. Jacob Zaun wrote: "In April of this year we took a girl . . . to live with us. She has a younger sister, now an inmate of the State Hospital for Crippled Children at Phalen Park. Her age is about twelve years. Since this

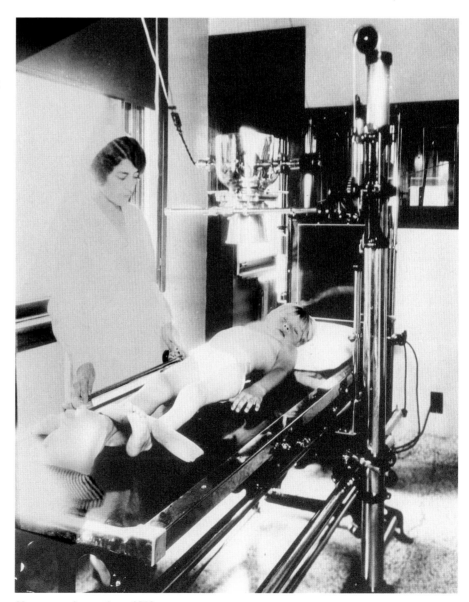

Nurse x-raying patient, 1930

43

girl came to us in April she has tried several times to visit her sister at Phalen Park, but the superintendent, a Mrs. McGregor, has refused to permit this. . . . I asked Mrs. McGregor why this girl was not allowed to visit her sister, and she informed me that it was impossible, as . . . she might bring in some infectious disease. What a ridiculous, yes even tragic, interpretation of a 'rule.' . . . A 'real' superintendent should be able to carry out the 'rules' in so far as this object is accomplished, but when the 'rules' defeat the object and inflict this unjustifiable, barbarous suffering on these poor children, [they] should be suspended or abrogated entirely." Miss McGregor did not find the restrictions on visitors ridiculous. She responded to the complaint in a letter to the State Board of Control: "I will say that the rule forbidding children to visit the hospital was adopted after whooping cough was brought in by the brother of a patient; the patient contracted it and later died."[12]

Diseases like measles, mumps, chickenpox, diphtheria, and smallpox were a constant concern. If possible, children with these conditions were sent to City and County Hospital, where they were placed in quarantine. Sometimes the number of children who were sick made this policy impossible to follow. During the two years of 1917 and 1918, 214 of the 426 children admitted to the hospital contracted one of these conditions. Quarantines of whole wards were common, and at times hospital admissions and visits were halted until an epidemic ran its course. The State Board of Control took the problem of communicable diseases seriously and published strict guidelines during the more severe outbreaks. During a smallpox epidemic in 1925, the board mandated that all hospital employees and visitors prove that they had been successfully vaccinated and required that the hospital post a guard at the door to keep out those not vaccinated. Vaccination was not a perfect solution. It was not unusual for adults to become sick after a vaccination, and the annual reports of the hospital often commented on the illnesses of the employees and their absences from work.[13]

By far the most serious epidemic in Minnesota during these years was the outbreak of Spanish

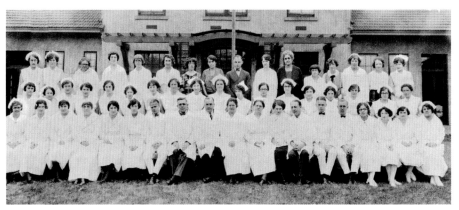

Nurses and staff, 1924

influenza. This devastating illness appeared abruptly in the fall of 1918 and spread throughout the entire state. From October 1918 through January 1919, 8,387 people died of influenza in Minnesota. In the decade before the epidemic, no more than 499 influenza deaths had occurred in any single year.[14] The young patients at the State Hospital for Indigent Crippled and Deformed Children were not spared. During the winter of 1918-1919, 125 children contracted influenza and many died. Particularly susceptible were the children with tuberculosis or other conditions which weakened their health. Dr. Carl Chatterton recalled how stressful the epidemic was for the doctors and nurses: "The flu epidemic in 1918 was a very serious situation because practically all our children who had tuberculosis and open sinuses who developed flu died. I remember I had a poor, young, house doctor, Dr. Brown, who met me one morning with tears in his eyes. He said, 'I can't take it, I've got to go home. I carried out four children last night. It gets me down. I just can't go on and work with children dying like that.'"[15]

Beginning in 1916, medical students and doctors still in training, known as interns or house doctors, were sent to the hospital by the University of Minnesota. Medical students attended clinics on Thursday mornings, and interns worked at the hospital for several weeks. During the 1920s four interns were assigned to the hospital at all times, and they were kept busy. They were expected to live

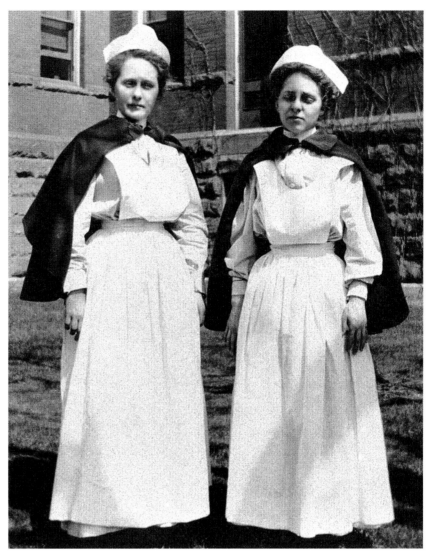

Nurses outdoors, circa 1911

there, and at least one was to be on duty at all times. When they left the campus they were required to register their departure and return in the office. Interns were expected to make rounds twice a day and to complete all dressing changes by 8 a. m. Interns also were responsible for obtaining a history of a newly admitted child's illness before the family left the hospital. A physical examination of each child was required, and after admitting a child, an intern was expected to administer vaccina-

tions and complete any necessary laboratory studies. Interns were not allowed to address nurses or employees by their first names and were not to "talk shop" during their meals in the dining room.

Some interns completed their tasks in an exemplary manner. Dr. Owen Wangensteen, later a famous surgeon and long-time chief of surgery at the University of Minnesota, received an "A" for effort as an intern in January 1922. Other interns chafed under the workload. Dr. Chatterton often had to write the university, as in this letter in 1924: "I am very anxious to learn from you the status of the University regulations concerning house doctors, as to their attendance upon service while in this institution. We repeatedly have our house doctors going out Saturday afternoon and not returning until Sunday night without informing us as to when they expect to return, or even asking permission. . . . We are perfectly willing to be reasonable and give the doctors as much time away as possible but it seems to me they have taken advantage. In my day when an intern absented himself over night the following day he was a candidate for dismissal from the institution." Thereafter the interns were given a written list of responsibilities.[16]

In the hospital's first thirty-one years, 4,750 children received care. Of those, 1,300 were described as cured, and 2,685 as improved. Although many of the hospital stays were long, and patients were away from their families, the children improved because the hospital brought together in one place all of the people who could help them. Much of the care was routine: good nutrition, good nursing, slow correction of deformities with casts, braces, and therapy, occasional surgeries, and education. Care was also creative. Tracings or pen and watercolor drawings of deformities were placed in patient records to serve as a baseline by which to judge the effects of treatment. Movies of some children were made as early as 1917. That year a child

was admitted, underwent surgery to lengthen a heelcord, and was discharged the same day. A child had a tendon lengthening performed with local anesthesia in 1924. Before intravenous administration of fluids became possible in 1924, fluids were given to surgical patients by injecting saline solutions into fatty tissues under the skin, or by placing large volumes of saline in the rectum so that it could be absorbed into the body. Transfusions of whole blood were done as early as 1927 and under anesthesia. Dental care began in 1916, and Novacaine was in use by 1919.

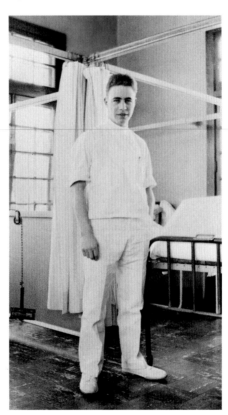

An intern, circa 1936

But there also were setbacks. Some medical care did not turn out well, and some seems unusual now. One child had a forceful

straightening of a badly deformed knee carried out under anesthesia. Blood flow to his foot was compromised and he developed gangrene. His life was saved by amputating his leg above the knee. Tonsillectomies were commonly done, sometimes in the hope of preventing outbreaks of diphtheria. One child developed massive swelling after a tonsillectomy and required a tracheostomy. The first lawsuit alleging poor medical care was filed in 1920 by a parent who believed that a cast had caused injury and permanent damage. The case was dismissed. X-ray treatments were given for whooping cough and skin lesions, mercury and arsenic were used to treat syphilis, and milk was sometimes injected into muscles to provide protein. On occasion, maggots were placed in sites of bone infection to remove pus and dead tissue.[17]

The hospital's experience was summarized in 1928. Of the first 4,750 children treated at the hospital, 312 were unchanged by their care, and 250 were still receiving treatment. Two hundred and three children had died while hospitalized, almost half of them from tuberculosis. Yet, there was much more to the story of the care they received than facts and figures and the annual reports of doctors and superintendents. A stay in the hospital left a deep impression on many children. Decades later, memories of their experiences were as alive as the days when they happened. When woven together, their stories tell us what children in the hospital saw and felt and how that changed their lives.

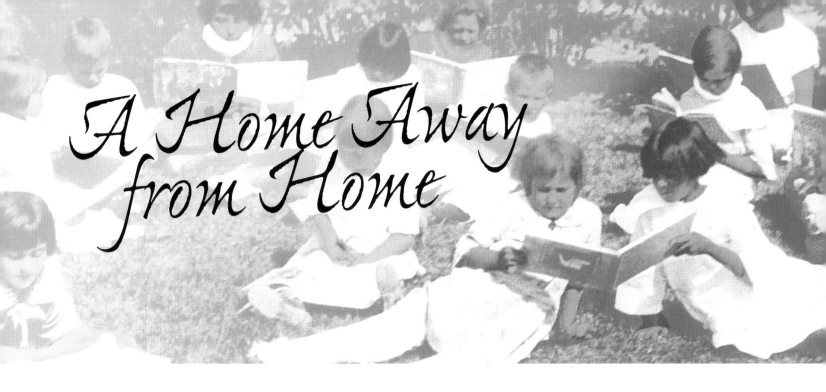

A Home Away from Home

In the 1920s Thursday was the day children were admitted to the hospital. Most of them were brought in by a parent, but some came with an aunt or an uncle or a public health official from their county. A few were placed on the train and met in St. Paul by a hospital employee or Miss McGregor. Almost all of the children remembered the low buildings with their tile roofs and the driving circle in front of the hospital.

The admission process was frightening and sometimes humiliating. The children were undressed, bathed, and their hair scrubbed to remove lice. The house officers obtained a history of the child's illness from family members and performed physical examinations, followed by laboratory tests and vaccinations. The examination room was large, and there was little privacy and little concern for the modesty of the children. Some of the children were isolated until it was certain they did not have an infectious disease. The departure of their parents was a wrenching experience, remembered years later by many children as a time of abandonment and intense loneliness until they made friends with other children in their ward.[1]

Daily life was ruled by the nursing staff. The nurses set the schedule, and as much as possible every event of the day was kept on time. Many of the nurses were loved. One of the most remarkable was Mary Wakefield. George Edmund Gilbertson, who was admitted in 1926 at two years of age and again in 1938 when he was fourteen, remembered her clearly. "In the vernacular of today, [he wrote in 1993] 'she was something else.' An even five foot tall, three foot at the beam, snowy white hair and then her little white cap and a white uniform . . . she looked like a little snowman, or should I say snow lady. . . . This lady pulled my hair, ears, and nose, and beat on my head with a spoon now and then. . . . She nursed me when I was ill, and punished me if she even suspected I had thought of doing something wrong, but she I loved more than all the rest put together."[2] Glenn Erickson, admitted in 1926 at age seven years old, also thought highly of Miss Wakefield: "She too was a jewel in my eyes. When

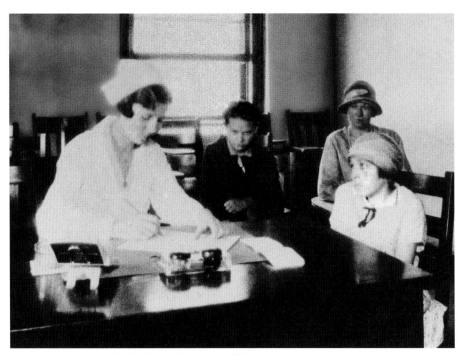

Admission to hospital, 1930 (see Appendix B)

necessary she would enforce rules with a loud voice and a twelve inch ruler. The ruler was waved in the air like an orchestra leader's baton, but it never found its way to the bottom of the problem." Other nurses left a positive memory. Glenn Erickson remembered two of them: "The word love today doesn't seem to have the same meaning as it did when it came to the staff at the hospital. In Ward One we had two very special nurses, Mrs. Carlson and Miss Tesch. Loving, caring, with a special attitude towards kids, they will never be duplicated. They made life worth living and took our minds off of our physical problems."[3]

A few of the nurses were despised. Mary Baehr described a nurse in her ward this way: "If the sun was shining in your eyes, do you suppose she'd pull a shade down? Not on your life. She just enjoyed seeing people suffer, I

think. She was abusive, to me. . . . For some reason or another there were some of the patients that she was mean to, and I was one of them. And finally one of them that she was mean to reported her

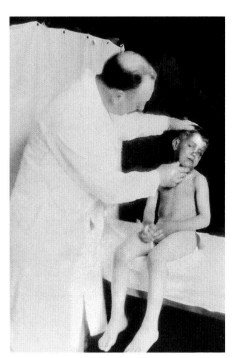

Patient examination, 1930

[to Miss McGregor] and you know, she was nice to me after that." Anne Carlsen described an encounter with another nurse: "Lights were out at nine and we were supposed to be quiet and go to sleep then, but that seldom happened. . . . [She] came in and told us we had no right to make a commotion because we were getting all this for nothing and we were too poor to be in a regular hospital. I reminded her that her job was being paid for by taxpayer money, too."

The children were grouped in large, segregated wards for boys and girls, with separate areas for the sickest children and those in isolation. For the most part the wards were organized by age groups, including a special ward for babies. The convalescent wards were the places where children made friends. As Glenn Erickson put it: "That was one of the best times of my stay at the

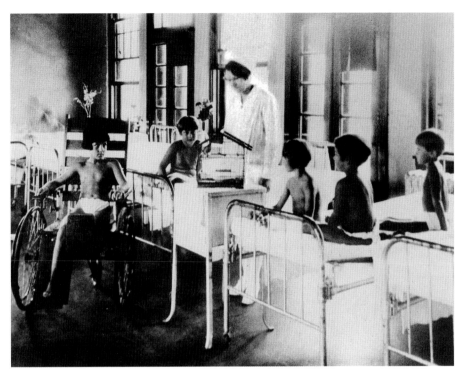

Nurse in ward with patients, circa 1930

hospital. Now I could go outside and play. Every boy in my ward was my best friend. We all had something in common, a bad leg here, a bad arm there." For some the ward was not as friendly. Bernie Pirjevec remembered that "there was an underworld, a 'bully system' with little boys who were slaves to the bigger ones."

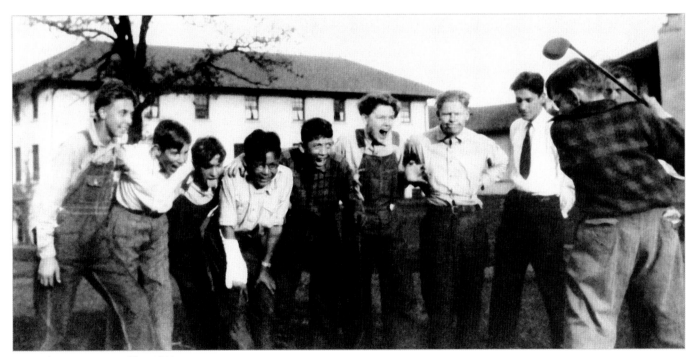

Boys cheering on a golfer, 1930

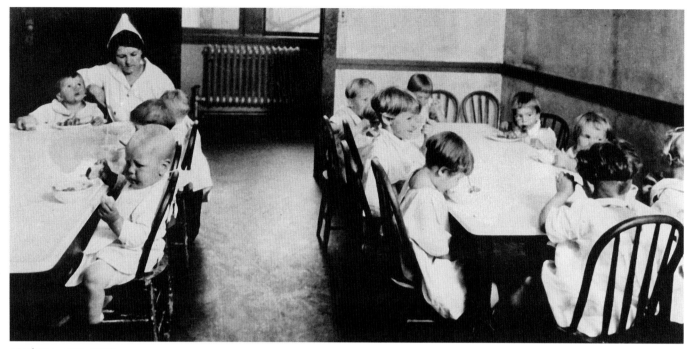

Mealtime, circa 1930

In every ward children were expected to help out with daily chores. Beds had to be made, and floors had to be swept. Some children needed help getting dressed. Berneil Nelson remembered that "I learned how to make up a very neat bed. The older girls were assigned ward tasks, and one was to line up all the beds in a perfect line and distance from each other on both sides of

I remember the swimming pool very much. I looked forward to having the casts taken off. I asked how soon I could be dumped in the swimming pool. They would wheel me in on a gurney with just a board top, and there would be attendants on the foot and head, and they would drop me in the pool. I never wanted to get out.

Mary Ellen (Mullaney) Radman
1994

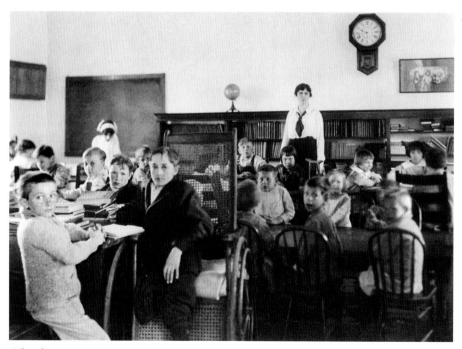

Schoolroom, circa 1920

the ward. We also swept floors. There was an inspection each day and if it wasn't right you did it again, especially on the days they expected the doctors to come through." In Ward Eight, a boy's ward, Miss Wakefield was quite particular about the beds. Joseph Baier remembered that "she would go down the middle of the aisle after you made the beds, and if there was anything wrong with it she pulled it all off on the floor and you had to make it all over. After she did it a couple of times we did it right."

The food left a big impression. Most of the children ate their meals in the dining room, a large room painted in bright pastel colors and populated by long dark wooden tables, each surrounded by ten chairs. Plates and bowls were stacked at one end of the table, and the silverware stood upright in holders at the center flanked by the salt and pepper shakers. The food was served in large bowls that were passed around the table. It was expected that any food placed on a plate would be eaten, and that when the bell rang to end the meal every plate would be clean. Many children remembered being required to eat vegetables and other undesirable things. Occasionally they were left to sit at their place until their plate was clean. Years later they still found it impossible to like beans, cauliflower, and spinach. Some of the children were quite creative in avoiding certain foods. Glenn Erickson was such a child: "Each day we lined up to march to the dining room. We had several long tables with a nurse at the head. Her job was to see that everyone cleaned their

> *One nurse forced me to swallow creamed peas, cheese and like foods at different times. I vomited each time. I can't stand the sight of such foods to this date.*
>
> **Bernie Pirjevec**
> **1993**

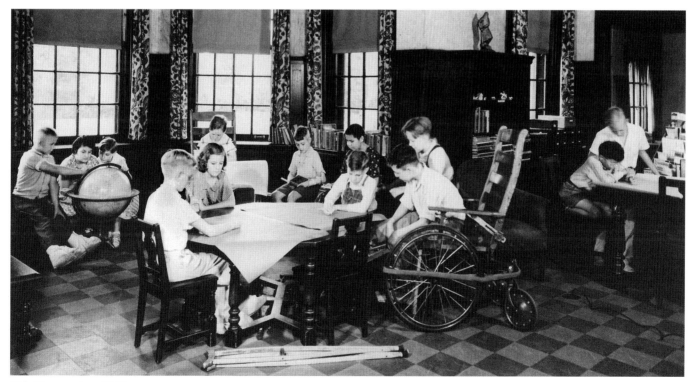

The library, circa 1945

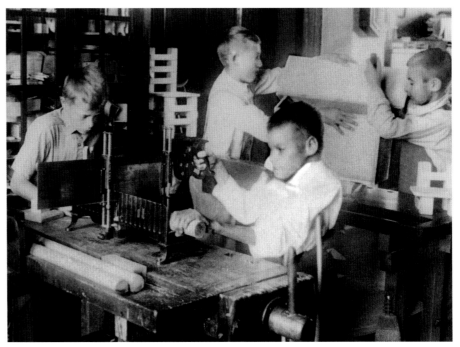

Woodworking class, circa 1930

plate. I could not stand to eat spinach, so in order to clean my plate I had to stuff the spinach in my pockets. On returning to my ward I would retire to our bathroom and flush spinach down the toilet. It was very messy but it served the purpose."

The daily routine included school and play. Education was a major focus, and classes were taught for children in grades one through twelve. Textbooks were purchased to provide a progressive curriculum, and examinations were given monthly to measure the progress of each student. Children restricted to their beds were given a half day of school work each day, and children who were able to be up spent five hours each day on their studies. By 1928 seven full-time teachers were employed. A library was created and became, as Miss McGregor put it, the "cultural center" of the hospital. Each child was required to attend four library periods each week, and story-tellers were very popular with the children.

An industrial school was created to give the children skills for everyday life. The skills taught reflected the expectations of the times. Girls learned sewing, cooking, and housekeeping. They made articles of clothing that were used on the wards. They used the kitchen to learn how to plan meals and reinforced their mathematical skills by planning budgets for a typical household. Boys were taught woodworking, basket weaving, and shop skills. They created toys and repaired furniture from the wards. They also worked in the gardens. Some of the projects were very successful. The girls entered clothing in competitions at the Minnesota State Fair. One year two of the boys won a birdhouse construction competition sponsored by a St. Paul newspaper. Another year the gardens at the hospital were named the best gardens in St. Paul.

Entertainment and play were important. A long list of citizens and social groups became involved with the hospital, contributing money, toys, fruit and candy, and entertainment. The Schubert Club gave concerts every other week during the winter. The Shriners transported children to the circus, and the Masonic women's groups provided clothing and gifts. Local theater groups gave performances and schooled the children in the production of short plays in which the children were the actors and actresses. Some of these productions attracted large audiences. Boy Scout and Girl Scout groups were formed, as was an Audubon club and a Junior Red Cross group. Day trips were a special treat. Each year children went to the State Fair by bus, to the state capitol for a

party given by state employees, and to Dr. and Mrs. Gillette's summer home near White Bear Lake for a picnic. A menagerie of pets was maintained, including rats, rabbits, guinea pigs, goats, dogs, cats, monkeys, ponies, donkeys, fish, and parrots. The children took care of some of the animals. On the hospital grounds there were sand boxes, swing sets, and a baseball diamond. Mysteriously, some of the children came back from outside play without their braces. Dr. Carl Chatterton told of a discovery made several years later. "Years ago we used to have a certain type of hip splint called a Sayer's hip splint. They were very uncomfortable to wear and the doctor would make rounds one morning and say 'Where's your splint?' and the poor little boy didn't know where the splint had gone. He hadn't seen it, and it was gone. But when they drained the little lake outside where

I remember Jack Dempsey, the boxer, came to entertain us in the auditorium. I still have his autograph.

**Eleanor (Hable) Weiss
1993**

I remember the time Rin Tin Tin, the dog, was brought in and he did tricks for us.

**Joan (Savage) Billison
1993**

I remember going to my first State Fair and having my first cup of coffee with cream. It was so good!

**Joan (Savage) Billison
1993**

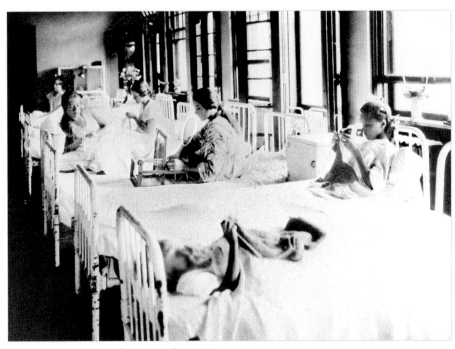

Knitting, weaving, and sewing class, 1930

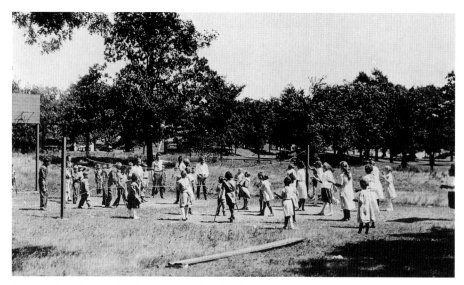

Girls against boys volleyball game, circa 1930

they built the new laundry I think they took 18 or 20 hip splints from the bottom of the lake."[4]

Life in the wards could be very interesting. The boys and girls were kept separate as much as possible, but they found ways to communicate. Alice Clancy remembered how hard it was to meet the boys: "Ward Six was boys and they were eight years old to sixteen years old. Of course we girls had eyes for them. We sent notes back and forth and one night we were supposed to meet them under the kitchen and the nurses got our note and so we girls were sitting up waiting for the boys and they never showed up." The children also taught each other games that the nurses did not appreciate. Joe Baier recalled learning to play poker: "I came from the country and did not know how to play poker, but a lot of these fellows knew how to play. They had to go to bed and they did not have any money, so they would play strip poker. Well, they got so that they did not have

any clothes on anymore and they still wanted to play, so they made other things they had to do. They had to run naked so many rows down the aisle and back again. I was the lookout. If we heard somebody coming we hollered and whoever was running would jump in the first open bed that he came to. The nurse knew where

everybody was and she knew that fellow was not in his bed. She would say 'You better get back to your bed.' She knew everything that was going on."

A series of parrots were residents in the wards, and they were very popular. The children were constantly teaching the birds words and phrases that annoyed the nurses. Glenn Erickson was in Miss Wakefield's ward: "She . . . had a very colorful parrot that was sitting on a perch by her desk. We were allowed to talk to the bird and teach it new words. One day the parrot said, 'damn it.' That was a dirty word at the time. She never found out who taught the bird to talk so bad, so it was off limits for quite some time." Some of the birds would tease and torment the children. One parrot developed the habit of watching for children returning to the ward from the recovery room after

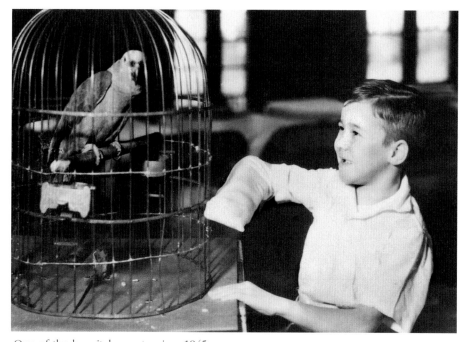

One of the hospital parrots, circa 1945

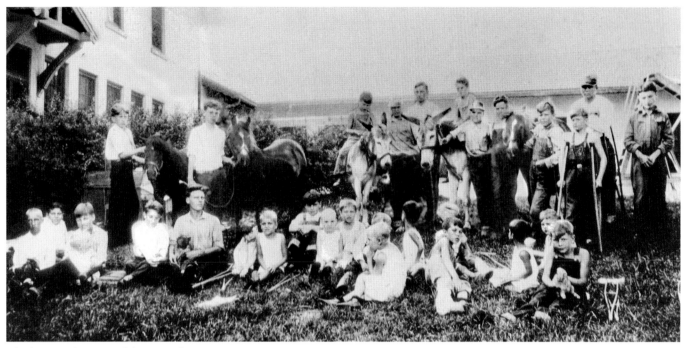

The boys with some of the animals, 1930

surgery. It would hop up on the overhead traction frame, look down on the child, and squawk, "bet it hurts, bet it hurts!" Some of the animals were more trouble than they were worth. This was true for the monkeys. Joe Baier told of one overactive monkey: "One time he got loose and across the street from the hospital was a college. I don't know what kind of college it was, but he got loose and went into a classroom where a class was being held. The teacher excused the class and the students took after the monkey and he came across the street and they got him in a corner. He bit one of the students, and then we couldn't have him anymore."

As happens with children, there were accidents and injuries. Some were serious, but most were minor events. One young man fell into the fish pond while playing ball. He was retrieved without

injury. One girl leaned too far out of a window and fell into the yard. Fights broke out every now and then, and the participants were punished by the nurses. Playing cards were a common cause of disputes, and Miss McGregor forbade card games for a time. Games with the animals sometimes caused injury. One boy was bitten by a monkey on two occasions, and several others were nipped by the parrots. Another child fell from one of the ponies while riding and broke his wrist. He stayed in the hospital a little longer until his wrist healed and his cast could be removed. Children also swallowed things, such as rubbing alcohol, keys, and whistles. Some of the more serious injuries were burns. The radiators were very hot in the winter, and several children fell against them and received burns. Miss McGregor wrote many letters to the State Board of Control and

I remember with fondness Dr. Chatterton driving onto the hospital grounds in his 1920 Franklin coupe. Air-cooled engine. Just think, no anti-freeze. He was a great doctor and a good guy.

**Chester (Weberg) Walker
1993**

There are over forty kids in this ward. At times there is as much noise as a boiler factory. We have some swell fights.

**Burton Aarness
1922**

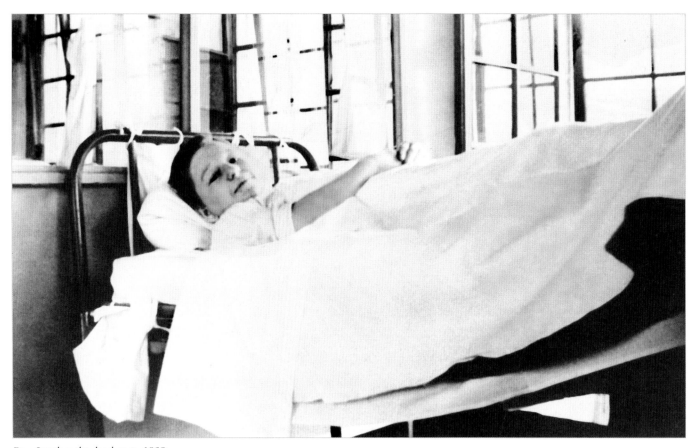

Rex Lambrecht, bed rest, 1939

the building contractors asking for protective coverings for the radiators. Hot plates were used in the wards, and on one occasion a nearby paper bag ignited, burning a chair and bed blankets before being extinguished. The child in that bed escaped injury. Another child was less fortunate; a steam inhaler tipped over and caused burns.[5] On occasion a child would sneak away from the grounds. Nearby stores were a favorite place to go. Elsa Hedberg remembered "trying to sneak out and go to the corner store to buy candy. The owner always reported us, and we would get a lecture from Miss McGregor."

The children were allowed a few personal possessions, which were kept in individual locked boxes. These boxes were the children's treasuries, a place where photographs, small toys, letters, and "stuff" could be kept. The items were put away each night, and each child kept a key on a string around his or her neck. Flashlights and yo-yos were very popular. Ed Gilbertson remembered how even a flashlight could become a toy. "The most important item in your box was more than likely your flashlight. At night, after lights out and after the nurse's footsteps faded, suddenly there on the ceiling would appear a spot of light as a sort of challenge. If there was no command to 'PUT THAT FLASHLIGHT AWAY' . . . the spot

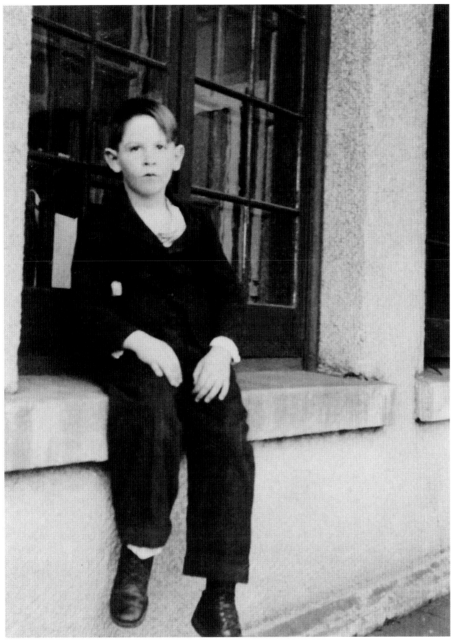

Young patient sitting on windowsill, circa 1930

nurses. Miss McGregor recognized that some children came from better circumstances than other children, and she worried that special gifts such as candy would cause trouble between the children. However, she was not insensitive. Joe Baier once received a package from his school at home. "Everyone [at the school] bought a candy bar and they put it in this box and they sent it to me. So, everybody got around me and I opened it up and here it was full of candy. Miss McGregor said 'No, you cannot have that,' and she shut it up and took it away. What happened was when the other patients left and were not around she said, 'You can come and have a candy bar when you are alone any time you want, but you have to eat it in the storeroom.' So I ate a whole box of candy in the storeroom. I was not supposed to let the other patients get suspicious of what I was doing."

On Thursday the doctors would make "grand rounds," traveling through the wards in a large group to examine and discuss the children. This left a big impression on the children. Joe Baier described it this way: "We would go to breakfast first and then we would come back and get undressed and put on a drape. That is when we would fight to get the biggest drape we could so that we would not be exposed. Miss McGregor would get all of the files out of the storeroom and put them on our beds. We would undress and lay down and wait for him.

would slowly circle and then suddenly shoot across the ceiling with another chasing it for all it could. Wow! Sometimes fifty beams would be running, waltzing, or just jumping for joy. . . . Suddenly, the overhead lights would snap on and there stood the night supervisor. . . . Down the line of beds came a nurse with

some container to collect all flashlights. They were confiscated for sometimes a week and would be returned with quite a speech."

The children cherished gifts that parents brought during visits or sent through the mail. A common gift was candy. In general gifts of food were not allowed, and candy usually was not approved by the

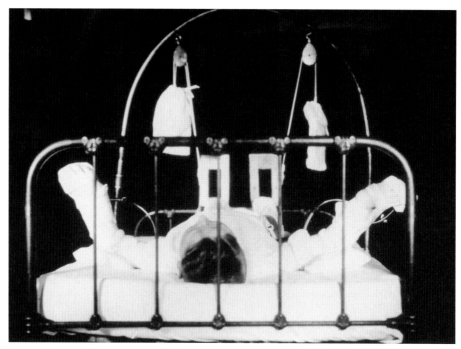

Arm splints and leg traction, 1936

Sometimes it would take quite a while. Some days . . . all he would do is tickle you on the bottom of the foot and keep on walking. After he left we had to get up again and dress and put everything away and put the beds in order and then we could go outside." Other Thursday visits were less pleasant. Ed Gilbertson was not fond of some of the house doctors: "Two had been my doctors from the beginning, and as they reached my bed I knew I was about to become a specimen of their learned pride . . . for if I was out of my armor each one of my arms and legs would be picked up, draped over a forearm, and the amount of movement would be shown. Now, these two guys were the best there were anywhere, and I had long before put my full trust in whatever they wanted to do, but, damn it, I would have just as soon those other yokels had kept their

mitts to themselves. For something like thirty years I had nightmares of one of them draping my stiff legs over his forearm and then, with the other, ramming the leg back to my butt."

The ward was a place where children could learn teamwork. Ed Gilbertson's story of revenge on a newspaper boy is a perfect example. "We had several paper boys over the years who, like any other boys had good and not too good sides. . . . The windows opened out onto the sidewalks of the hospital, and many of them, who weren't scared of us, would drape over the sills and talk to us. . . . There was one boy who was just mean through and through. Never did he have a good word for anyone. . . . This newsboy would at times gather a handful of grass and weeds, with dead and not so dead insects, and as he walked by he would make sure no one was watching and, as my head was toward the window and I was in full arms reach, he would reach in and cover my face with whatever goodies he had selected for his pleasure. . . . The attack that infuriated me the most came during a hot spell in July or August. With the temperature in the nineties and the humidity near the same, and me in full armor, he waltzed up to the window and with careful aim let go with a mouth full of water he had carried for three blocks just for this purpose. Not only was it hot but it was slimy from his saliva. Then, to add insult to it, there was no way I could reach my face to wipe and I had to lay there and wait for it to dry. . . . [The other children] left it to me to pick our revenge. A few days went by before a plan to everyone's liking was okayed

and put into play. Everyone wanted to be in on this one. So, on the day our plan was executed my bed was pushed away from the window far enough for Ralph to hide on the floor. As soon as we saw the kid coming we were set. It took us awhile to convince him there were no hard feelings and that I really wanted a paper. Greed overcame doubt, and when he reached for my money Ralph's arm shot up and caught his shirt front. Then came the coup d'etat. Ralph was handed a full urinal, which all twelve of us had helped to fill. He pushed the kid's head back out the window and, without loosening his grip, slowly poured every drop over his head. Papers flew in all directions and the kid was screaming at the top of his lungs. . . . Our little party had not attracted a single nurse

or anyone, so we spent the afternoon living it over and over."

Ed Gilbertson was also present when a tornado struck, one of the most frightening hospital events in the 1920s. "The blue sky . . . turned the most sickening cold yellow ever seen. About this time I noticed that a few of the nurses appeared from nowhere, stationing themselves at different locations in the ward, with one in the doorway near my bed. . . . It got so dark you just knew it couldn't get any darker. There was a pause, and then every window in the ward imploded at once, sending glass everywhere. Then came the wind and the rain sweeping horizontally through the windows, ripping off my top sheet. . . . I let out a scream . . . and without hesitation fifty voices joined me. The poor nurse was caught unprepared and . . . grabbed me . . . and shook me so hard I was beginning to see two sheets for every one in the air. Suddenly, she dropped me . . . and hurried off to help the others. I was so angry at her for shaking me that I wouldn't speak to her for two days. . . . The end of the second day she came over to . . . ask forgiveness. She squeezed my right index finger, and said 'please.' That squeeze on the finger was the only sign of affection I ever received in the hospital."

Still, affection was present, and came from very different people. Ed Gilbertson's birthday was December 28, and his mother always came to visit. One year the birthday visit was not possible. Ed remembered how the day was

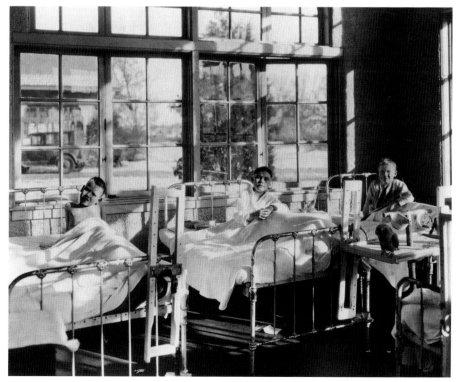

Boys in their beds on the porch and a parrot on it's perch, circa 1930

saved: "My mother was unable to get down to see me and wrote to Miss McGregor. . . . This very busy lady not only took the time to come out of her office and tell me, but she stopped by the kitchen and had them bake a whole sheet cake, enough so that every one of the fifty kids in Ward Five had a big piece of Ed's Birthday Cake. I don't think that birthday has ever been topped."

Ed Gilbertson also learned something from Hannah, a cleaning woman who worked in his ward. "I saw Hannah nearly every day of my young life, but I don't think that in all those years fifty words passed between us, though we were often within three feet of one another. I think it was she who taught me patience and sticking with something once having started. There was nothing pretty or attractive about her, I'm sorry to say. She was tall and gangly, with long dark hair laced with gray and pulled back tightly without a part. It was tied on the back of her head in a straggly bun. Her eyes were sunk deeply into her skull, with high, protruding cheekbones.

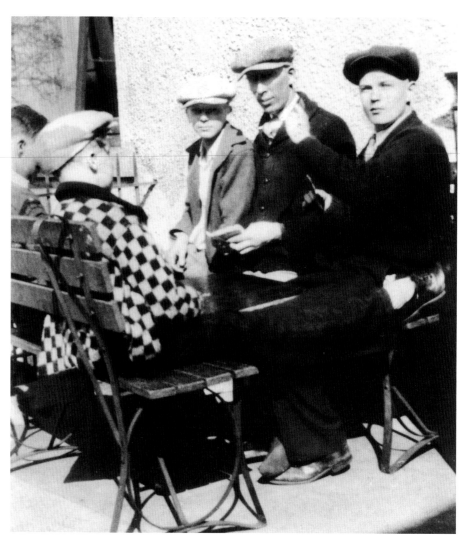

Playing cards outside Ward Six, 1929

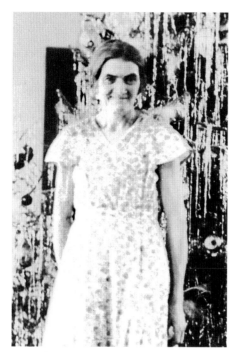

Hannah, a janitress, circa 1932

There was not an ounce of fat on her face or any part of her body. She had very few teeth in her mouth, and they only served to make her look sinister. No one ever talked to her unless it was to tell her to clean up the mess some kid had barfed over the edge of his bed. I know not what nationality she was, but she had very dark skin. I knew her to be a good person because if my mother happened to be visiting the two of them would move over towards the windows and speak to each other for a few minutes. Every so often Hannah would lean way over on her mop and ask me how I was feeling that day. I was scared, but due to mother's judgment of her I felt pretty safe. . . . It was years before I learned why every so often she would lean on her mop and a most pleasant smile would appear at the corners of her mouth. Then one day . . . my

bed was aligned just right when that smile appeared and I quickly looked to see . . . and there it was, all laid out for me. Hannah had come down the wide aisle the length of the ward with this wide figure-of-eight sweep of her mop. The loops on each side were perfect, and none had overlapped. The whole pattern of probably sixty feet was perfect. Then she leaned on her mop handle, and we watched the pattern fade without one single line drying before the other. Like magic it disappeared, leaving no trace. She looked away and our eyes happened to meet. I smiled, one of my best, and she knew I had witnessed the event and understood it."

The holiday season of Thanksgiving and Christmas was a sad, and a happy, time. Every child hoped to be home for Christmas, but every year dozens of children had to stay in the hospital for the holiday. Years later many of those children held strong memories of Christmas in the hospital. Every ward had a decorated tree, and a special meal was served. Community groups showered the hospital with gifts for the children, and Santa Claus came to distribute them. Mary Baehr remembered how the staff tried to make the day special: "They used to take up a collection for the toys for [the hospital]. And so we were all supposed to write a letter to Santa Claus requesting three gifts. We'd get what we asked for. They tried hard to get what we wanted." The children sang carols, and community groups put on skits. Occasionally

Dear Folks, I'll try my hand at a letter tonight. . . . I'll write of Christmas. Sunday night we hung our stockings. I opened mine when temperatures were being taken around three o'clock. We got an apple, a popcorn ball, and a box of five chocolate candies. Monday we were up early. We waited around until nine o'clock when a Santa from downtown came and gave out the presents. From the hospital fund I received a book of poems, chessmen and a chess board, and a knife. . . . After the kids received their stuff there was a disorderly house. Toys were broken and thrown away galore. Alvin Berg and I were in the bathroom and salvaged a few things.

**Burton Aarness
1922**

The only place that I felt normal and felt good about myself was when I was in the hospital.

**Mary (Bazzachini) Baehr
1993**

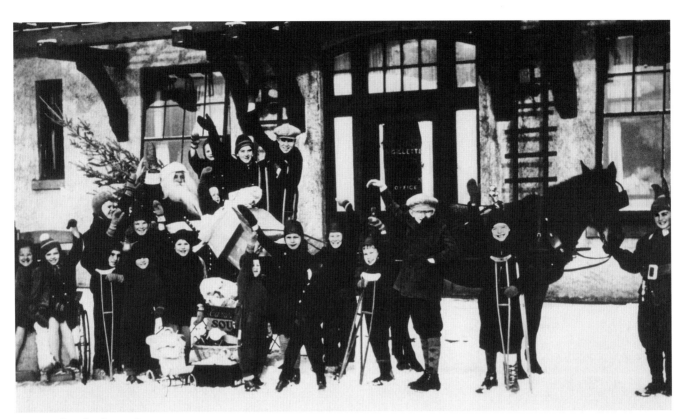

Santa in his sleigh, 1925

the entertainment was unplanned. One year the staff dressed a pony as a reindeer and had him pull a sled through the wards. The "reindeer" pooped on the floor.

Special acts of kindness by nurses on Christmas were long remembered. One year Ed Gilbertson and the boys in his ward were given a special gift by a young nurse. "That year there was a nurse whose face and name has slipped my memory but never will I forget her. The tree had been trimmed for a few days, and we were thrilled with it. Then, about two hours before her shift was over, she came into the ward with a shopping bag filled with tree trimmings. She walked around and let us choose one. I was in my armor that year so she chose a sparkling bunch of tinsel and put it in my right hand. Then this little lady went back to the first bed, pulled it from its place, and ran the length of the ward with it. She skid to a stop and then moved the bed in so that the kid could hang the trimming he had chosen. She went back to each and every bed, and for two hours she ran that floor and gave each of us the same thrill ride. I was in the last bed . . . and the anticipation of the ride had made me so excited that my tinsel had become nothing more than a sweaty handful of tinsel that resembled a shiny bird's nest. She grabbed the bed, spun it out to the middle of the floor, and started to run. . . . It took my breath away. We reached the tree and found just the right spot for a bird's nest. I couldn't reach so I asked her to place it for me so that I could see it from my last bed in the row. When she realigned my bed she stepped to the middle of the doorway, still smiling, bowed and quietly walked out. . . . The next morning when she walked in we were ready. At the top of our voices we gave our 'One, two, three, four, who are we for? Five, six, seven, eight, who do we appreciate,' and a big 'hooray.' Though she didn't say anything, I'm sure she noticed that there wasn't a wrinkle in the covers of any bed, and they stayed that way for her full shift. . . . Except for changing dressings and taking temperatures she had no real duties that day and spent every moment she could leaning at the foot of our beds, talking to us. At the end of the day she stood in the doorway again and very quietly thanked us."

Every child longed for the day on grand rounds when the doctors would say, 'time for you to go home.' Alice Meland remembered waiting for the magic words from her doctor: "We all counted the days and hoped the doctor would say we could go home, but no one ever got to go home in only six weeks. I prayed and prayed to God to let me go home." Yet, for some children, it was hard to go home. Alice Clancy described the paradox: "I cried when I had to go [to the hospital] and had to see my parents go, but after I was there I was fine. And then, when I got home, I cried because I wanted to go back." At home the children were different from other children. Glenn Erickson described one useful aspect of being in the hospital: "The good part of these four years of my life was that we were all equal. Nobody stared at us, nobody whispered about us, nobody was sorry for us. The bad part was going home to normal people." Sometimes the long separation from family was the problem. Mary Baehr was hospitalized ten times between 1921 and 1935: "I had to be away and I never really knew my mother and father. And, I never really knew my brothers and sisters. I just felt like a stranger when I came home." Berneil Nelson came to understand the cost of separation from her family: "I missed all the family gatherings and events at home. My sister talks about people and things

happening that I don't remember at all, most likely because I wasn't there." Glenn Erickson put it simply: "I cried for my pals in [the hospital]. We had something, we had everything in common."

What the children held in common was the ability to see

more than crooked backs and arms and legs, or braces and crutches and wheelchairs. Occasionally a visitor looked past these things, too. In 1974 Gareth Hiebert wrote about Dora and Arthur Larsen in a column in the *St. Paul Pioneer Press*:

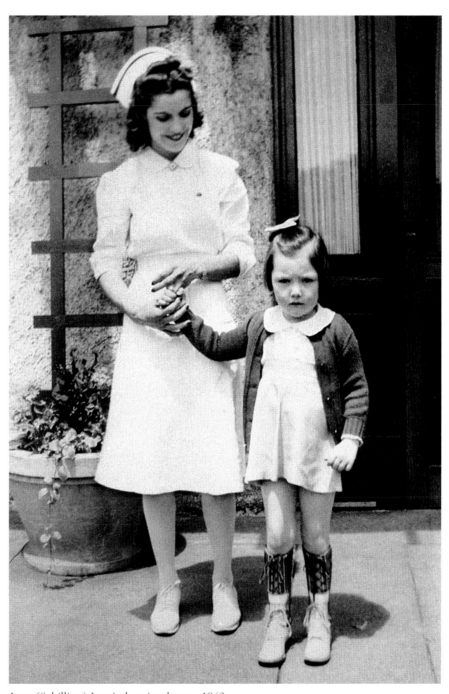

Jean (Schilling) Legried, going home, 1942

She was 18. He was 28. . . . She was a patient, a victim of polio since the age of four. . . . He was strong, tall. And he came to visit his sister who lay in the next bed. . . . Dora saw him and smiled. He smiled back. Her heart missed a beat. He says now that his did, too. She thought: "Who would ever want to marry a girl like me, who will never walk properly and may end up in a wheel-chair?" It crossed his mind, but not his heart.

Dora had undergone several operations performed by Dr. Gillette and Dr. Chatterton and was recovering from another surgery when she met Arthur. Hiebert recounted how they met:

"I lay there waiting for my Prince Charming to come along." "Instead she got me," Arthur always breaks in at this point. She squeezes his hand and says: "Oh, he was my Prince Charming all right. Why, I used to hobble down the hall to meet him for dates in the dark corners."

They fell in love and after Dora went home to Truman, Minnesota, Arthur knew he wanted to marry her. He went to visit her and proposed. They were married in a preacher's home on Christmas Eve in 1924 and had three children. Dora told Hiebert about the challenges of raising children:

I guess my children understood from the time they could comprehend that I was a little different from other mothers. . . . I only said, "No!" to them once and they knew I couldn't afford to say it again. . . . [There were] times when I'd worry where they had got to and I couldn't run to help them as fast as other mothers . . . times my husband had to be both father and mother. . . . But, I never let them pity me once, nor did they use the word cripple.

Hiebert's article was written on the occasion of Dora and Arthur Larsen's fiftieth wedding anniversary party, but Dora refused to make it all seem so wonderful and perfect.

I won't say we've lived always happily or without tensions, sorrow, sacrifice, disappointments . . . but if I hadn't seen him and he hadn't looked at me twice . . . none of you would be here to listen to the Christmas Eve story and get stuffed on my cooking.

Hiebert concluded his article with this observation: "It is odd that if Dora Gaston had never gotten polio, Arthur Larsen would never have met her. That's how she thinks. . . . Someone is sure to want to help push Dora's wheelchair and Arthur will come over and say 'here, let me do it. I've had some experience.' He will look at her, and she at him, and they'll laugh with love for each other."[5]

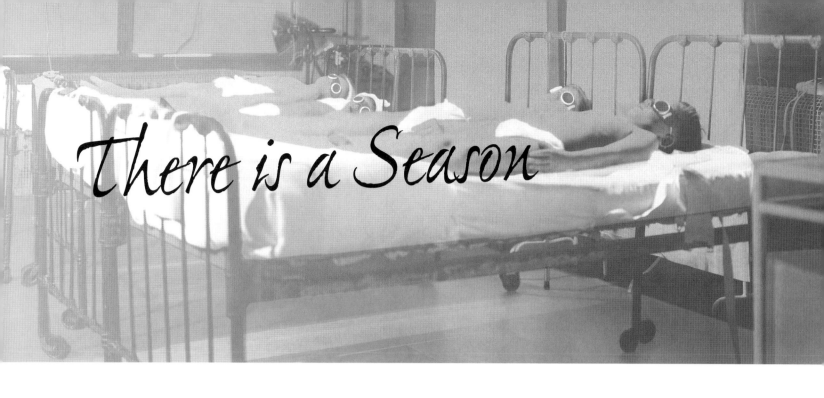

There is a Season

With the hospital settled at Lake Phalen, the 1920s witnessed the passing of the people who had formed it. In the span of eleven years, Arthur Gillette, Jessie Haskins, Michael Dowling, Arthur Ancker, and Stephen Mahoney were all gone. Their places were filled by Elizabeth and Margaret McGregor, Carl Chatterton, and Wallace Cole.

In 1898 a reporter for the *Minneapolis Journal* had described Arthur Gillette as "a very busy man."[1] That was an understatement. In addition to his service at the hospital for crippled children, he maintained a busy private practice at his office in the Moore Building in the Seven Corners area of St. Paul. He sent his adult patients to several St. Paul hospitals including City and County Hospital, St. Luke's, St. Joseph's, and Bethesda. He published numerous scholarly papers on orthopaedic topics, and gave dozens of talks. In 1900 Gillette was a member of the Editorial and Publication Committee for the first two volumes of *The St. Paul Medical Journal.* He belonged to several medical societies, where he was well-liked and respected. In 1896 he was elected president of the Ramsey County Medical Society, and in 1900 he became president of the American Orthopaedic Association, the oldest national professional society for orthopaedic surgeons in the United States. He also was elected president of the Minnesota Academy of Medicine in 1907 and president of the Minnesota Medical Association in 1917.[2]

Gillette was first appointed to the medical faculty of the University of Minnesota in 1895, when he was made an instructor in orthopaedic medicine. In 1897 he was promoted to clinical professor; in 1898, at the suggestion of Dr. James Moore, he was made a full professor with the right to vote in faculty meetings. In 1903, in recognition of his many contributions to the university, he was given an honorary medical degree. In 1915, when the regents reorganized the department of surgery, a division of orthopaedic surgery was created, and Gillette was placed in charge. A year later the medical school made the hospital for crippled children at

Phalen a regular site for the education of medical students, interns, and house officers.[3]

In 1890 Gillette married Ellen Moore, and they lived at 301 Pleasant Avenue, St. Paul. They had one child, Margaret, who married Vincent O'Brien and also lived in St. Paul at 1149 Summit Avenue. Ellen Gillette died in 1905 at the age of forty of pernicious anemia. Two years later, Gillette married Katherine Kennedy, who had been a teacher at the hospital for crippled children when it was located at City and County Hospital. They had no children. Their summer home in Dellwood was a frequent site for summer picnics for children from the hospital.[4]

Dr. Gillette's health began to fail noticeably in 1918. He had been a vigorous man, and Frederic Norton's description of him in 1899 was typical: "Dr. Gillette . . . was a portly man, of medium height, with a pleasant face. He did not waste words, was direct and to the point, was rather gruff, but had a heart as big as all outdoors."[5] In 1917 Gillette volunteered for military service but was not accepted because of a heart condition. By late 1918 he had reduced his office hours, and in early 1919 friends noticed that he had lost weight and tired easily.

Dr. Arthur J. Gillette, circa 1910

Finally, he left Minnesota for most of the winter of 1919–1920.[6]

In anticipation of the hospital's twenty-fifth anniversary in 1922, or perhaps sensing that Dr. Gillette was dying, Elizabeth McGregor began to contact former patients and others who had been involved in the start of the hospital. In January and February 1920, she wrote dozens of letters, most of them similar to the letter she sent to the hospital's very first patient:

We are anxious to know how everyone who has ever been at the State Hospital are at this time. We will appreciate it very much if you will write, giving us any information about your health, or any other information such as the line of business you are in, whether you have a family, and anything of a personal nature that you may think will be of interest. We would like very much to have Dr. Gillette see all the old patients, but this may be impossible. We will be glad to hear from you.

Jessie Haskins received one of those letters. On February 28, 1920, Miss McGregor asked Jessie to write a short autobiography, describe her involvement in the creation of the hospital, and send a picture of herself. Jessie responded promptly, for on March 16, Miss McGregor wrote to thank her. Unfortunately, the autobiography,

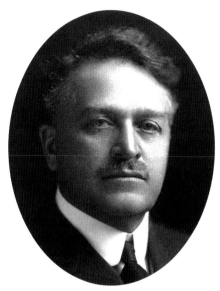

Dr. Arthur J. Gillette, circa 1920

the hospital history article, and the photograph all have been lost.[7]

In October 1920 Miss McGregor commissioned William Churchill, a well-known Boston artist, to paint Dr. Gillette's portrait while Churchill was in St. Paul to complete another work. He finished the portrait on November 17, 1920, and delivered it to the hospital the week after Thanksgiving. Churchill charged $900 for the portrait and arranged to have a gilded, carved frame measuring forty by fifty-five inches built by a firm in Boston at a cost of $97.80. In December 1920 Miss McGregor organized a small party at the hospital to unveil the portrait, which then was displayed on a wall near the hospital's offices. Within a month Dr. Gillette's health had begun to deteriorate rapidly.

On March 22, 1921, he suffered a stroke while at his daughter Margaret's home. He fell into a coma and died the next day.[8]

The love his friends had for him became clear in letters published in newspapers and medical journals, and in the memorial written about him at the University of Minnesota. The first editorial comment came in *The Journal-Lancet,* on April 1, 1921.

The determined seriousness into which mankind has been plunged is teaching us things which we only vaguely guessed before. We are becoming conscious of death, and of sacrifice and usefulness which we did not know existed. We are withstanding tests and rising to heights of achievement of which we did not think ourselves capable, and we are discovering potentialities which we might never have learned. Certainly under the stress of the present conflict something greater than ourselves has taken hold of us and uplifted us, and in our suffering and seriousness many great lessons of life have been borne in upon us. For the past few years America has grown up, as it were. As a nation she has been confronted with gigantic problems; she has been baptized by dangers and tribulations. . . .

After the war doctors will know by actual experience that it requires knowledge, scientific skill and experience to build a hospital. They will learn that a hospital is not simply brick, mortar and stone and a few saintly pictures. . . .

One of the greatest things this war is going to bring about, both abroad and in America, will be to accentuate the part a woman can fill in this world, the part which she has so justly claimed and fought for for many years. . . . She will demonstrate a woman can be just as good a doctor or surgeon as a man. . . .

We all make mistakes more than we should because of hurried examinations and incomplete records. . . .

It will teach us that the surgeon, who is the operator, must have assistance and be told when and where to operate; to know this is very often far more important than to be the operator. . . .

After this war there will be no place for pseudo-scientific, camouflage medicine-men. . . .

Already you will observe from the character of the various articles that are appearing in our medical journals, that we are becoming more and more interested and realizing more and more the importance and necessity of conservation of life, beginning in early life.

Dr. Arthur Gillette, Presidential Address
Minnesota State Medical Association, 1918

As *The Journal-Lancet* is choosing its forms for the press, word comes from St. Paul that Dr. Arthur J. Gillette is dead—dead at the age of fifty-seven. Dr. Gillette's monument has already been erected in his years of devotion to crippled children and especially in the Phalen Park State Hospital for such unfortunates, which was the first institution of its kind in America. He will long live lovingly in the memories of those children—thousands of them—and their parents and relatives. But his beneficences went far beyond those treated by him or under his direction. His scientific work made it possible for orthopedic surgeons the world over to do better work, and to alleviate suffering in its keenest form. His monument stands foursquare to the world, and if there be written upon three sides of it memorials to his scientific worth as a physician and surgeon, the fourth side shall be reserved for a testimonial to the manly man—manly in all the relations of life.[9]

The profound respect for Gillette's human qualities came through in the words of Emil Geist and R.O. Beard. Geist, an orthopaedic colleague, remembered Gillette as "a real and lovable man." Beard, secretary of the University of Minnesota Medical School faculty, placed Gillette's personal qualities first in the faculty memorial published in *Minnesota Medicine.*

Success comes to many, as it came to him; but success with distinction is won, as he won it, by few. The genial nature, the kindly humor, the punctilious courtesy, the careful professionalism, like the diagnostic fingers and the analytic mind of the man, were peculiarly his own. There was a strong personal quality in everything he did which made for the large sum of appreciation he received from his fellows.

The tendency to give Gillette exclusive credit for the creation of

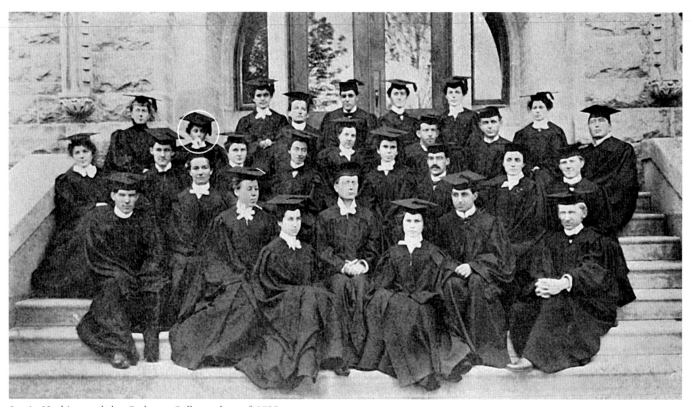

Jessie Haskins and the Carleton College class of 1899

the hospital for crippled children reached its peak in Beard's words.

> The one great ambition of his life, The Hospital for Crippled and Deformed Children at Phalen Park, the first institution of its kind in America, stands as his personal and professional monument. He conceived it, he inspired the gift of the acreage upon which it stands, he framed and promoted the legislation which created it, he superintended its construction, he directed its activities throughout its history, he determined that its staff should be of the university faculty. A model of its kind, a noble institution of the State, an educational asset of the University, it has been, under his inspiration, more than all of these, a place of light and leadership, of human love and human service.

Beard found the essence of Arthur Gillette.

> Service was the keynote of the life of Arthur Gillette; his one great purpose was to promote the happiness of the handicapped. The smiles and the laughter of little children whose lives he lengthened, whose sufferings he assuaged, whose deformities he corrected, whose health he restored, whose usefulness and satisfaction he assured, will be his welcome in the world to which he has gone, as they

were the light and the music of the world he has left.[10]

In 1925 a bill was introduced in the legislature to change the name of the Minnesota State Hospital for Indigent Crippled and Deformed Children to Gillette State Hospital for Crippled Children. Widely supported, the bill was backed by the State Board of Control. As one board member put it, "In view of the fact that he did more to bring about the establishment of the hospital than anyone else in Minnesota, and that he gave his services to it free of charge from the time it was started until his death, the members of the board feel it would be very appropriate to have the institution bear his name." The bill passed unanimously.

There is no record of Jessie Haskins's response to Gillette's death. After the struggle with the legislature in 1897 to create the hospital, Jessie returned to her studies at Carleton College. She graduated on June 14, 1899, along with thirty other students in her class, with a bachelor of literature degree. The sketch of Jessie in the Carleton College yearbook for 1899 showed the respect she had earned from her classmates.

> Jessie Alice Haskins is one of our thinking, self-reliant members who does not depend upon other people for opinions. She was the only free silverite in the class, and was an ardent supporter of all Bryan's doctrines. Although she has announced

> *Dr. Gillette died on March 23rd. He was in bed one day but had been very poorly all winter. Mr. Churchill painted his portrait last fall. . . . I do not think the portrait is a good one but we are very glad to have it and glad it was done while he could realize it.*
>
> **Elizabeth McGregor**
> **1921**

> *His lofty ideals, unselfish motives and constant friendship won him early and wide recognition as a leader in his chosen specialty. He will be long remembered by all with whom he came in contact, both for his gentle and considerate kindness and for his professional attainments.*
>
> **Drs. Wallace Cole, Robert Earl, and C. E. Riggs**
> **1921**

that her aim in life is to work as little as possible, those who know her best know that she left an artist's life for one of prosaic college duties. When she returns to her home on the Columbia, we feel sure that her gift for story writing, which has already been recognized, will win for her a prominent place among writers of fiction.[11]

Jessie returned to Spokane to live with her mother. The 1899 Spokane Directory recorded the occupation of Laurena C. P. Haskins as journalist; she lived at E1555 North River Avenue. The 1900 Directory showed that Jessie and her mother had moved to E1911 North River Avenue. In 1901 they were joined by Ella, whose husband Arthur had died. The 1900 United States Census listed Jessie as a single woman who could read, write, and speak English, and her occupation was listed as an author. By 1903 the Directory listed her as a teacher.

On June 8, 1904, Laurena Haskins died of paralysis, which may well have been the result of a stroke. She was buried in Greenwood Cemetery, and on the monument her daughters erected was carved a passage from scripture: "Her children shall rise up and call her blessed." Shortly before their mother's death, Jessie and Ella moved to E2309 Illinois Avenue in Spokane, and they lived there the rest of their lives. Jessie never married. From 1905 to 1910, she was employed at the Spokane Public Library,

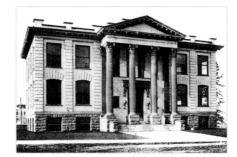

Spokane Public Library, circa 1910

working in the circulation and registration department.[12]

We know little more of Jessie's life after she moved to Spokane. She seems to have fallen silent after her advocacy for crippled children during her years at Carleton. A story Jessie wrote in 1897 for *The Carletonia,* the college's literary publication, gives hints at how she saw herself. The story was set in Tacoma, Washington, and tells of Dorothy, a young lieutenant in the Salvation Army, and her encounters with two men. One is a captain in the Salvation Army and good in every way. The other, John Ellwood, is wealthy, undisciplined, and faithless.

The story opens with a description of the city and moves to the scene of a raucous group of men leaving a theater. A Salvation Army group, which includes Dorothy, is marching up the street and confronts the men. One of them, the well-to-do young John Ellwood, becomes caught up in the Salvation Army speeches and is fascinated by Dorothy and her speeches.

One evening Ellwood is sitting in a carriage when the noise of another confrontation frightens his horse, and the carriage crashes into the Salvation Army marchers, severely injuring Dorothy. Ellwood accompanies her to the hospital with the Salvation Army captain and obtains a specialist for her. A slow recovery follows, and Ellwood realizes how much he cares for Dorothy. He visits her with the young captain, and sees that this man is also fond of Dorothy, and she of him. As the captain reads from Psalm 121, Dorothy takes a convalescent

The Lord Our Protector

121 I look to the mountains
Where will my help come from?

My help will come from the Lord, who made heaven and earth.

He will not let you fall; your protector is always awake.

The protector of Israel never dozes or sleeps.

The Lord will guard you; he is by your side to protect you.

The sun will not hurt you during the day, nor the moon during the night.

The Lord will protect you from all danger; he will keep you safe.

He will protect you as you come and go now and forever.

Psalm 121 from the book of *Psalms.*

toddler from the children's ward into her arms and plays with him. Ellwood realizes he is in love with her, only to hear her repeat the Psalm verse, and die.

This sentimental Victorian story suggests Jessie's outlook on life in its portrayal of a young, energetic, and vocal woman who holds strong moral beliefs. The young woman is badly injured and never fully recovers. That also was Jessie's fate. Ella (Haskins) Holly observed years later that Jessie was sensitive about her spine curvature and that curvature changed her image of herself, perhaps making her self-conscious and uncomfortable in relationships with other people. It also limited her activities. As Ella said, the curve "caused her much suffering in childhood, and great mental distress as well, as she grew older and realized that she could not do many of the things which she would have loved to." Jessie's shoulder injury, the result of a fall from a horse, only made her burden worse.

We do not know if Jessie's health, or her melancholy about her curvature, played a role in her remaining single. In addition to her work at the Spokane Public Library, she continued her efforts as a writer. In 1911 Jessie and Ella, writing under pseudonyms, wrote a novel entitled *The Man with the Scar*. The book was published by Gorham Press of Boston.[13]

In February 1927, F. H. Haggard of the Carleton College alumni office received a letter from Maude Spear, a member of the class of 1899. In her letter, dated February 11, she told Haggard that she had received that day a letter from Martha Ann Fischer, a classmate, reporting that Jessie had died. Fischer wrote that on or about February 11, Jessie had suffered "an attack of weakness of the heart, and on Monday, February 14, fell quietly asleep and slipped into that Better Land where there is no more sorrow or tears." It is reasonable to assume that Maude Spears, Martha Ann Fischer, and Jessie Haskins were friends. All three had received bachelor of literature degrees when they graduated in 1899.[14]

Her information, however, was not accurate. According to her death certificate, Jessie became ill on February 6 and died at home at 1:30 on the afternoon of February 7. The cause of death was "acute dilatation of the heart." Most likely this was heart failure, perhaps following a heart attack. She was sixty-one years old and the first of her sisters to die. The spine curvature of her childhood may well have contributed to her death. Severe curves of the spine twist and distort the rib cage. This, in turn, reduces the space for the lungs, and makes the heart work harder. Death comes early as the heart and lungs grow tired from their effort.

The public took little notice of Jessie's death. No editorials were written, and no memorials were published. The only mention of her role in the creation of a hospital that had improved the lives of thousands of children was a brief obituary published in the Spokane newspaper, *The Spokesman-Review*, on the day of her funeral.

> Through an accident in childhood, Miss Haskins had always been deprived of the activity of a child. For that reason, she had taken a great interest in unfortunate children. While she was a student at Carleton College, Minnesota, where she graduated thirty years ago, she succeeded in getting through the state legislature of Minnesota, virtually by her own efforts, a bill providing for a state hospital for crippled children.

The newspaper received its information from Ella. After the funeral, Jessie's body was cremated. Her ashes were buried next to her mother, and the site was marked with a simple, flat stone that reads: Jessie Alice Haskins, 1866-1927, Daughter of H. D. and L. C. P. Haskins.[15]

On April 21, 1921, only a month after the death of Arthur Gillette, Michael Dowling died at St. Luke's Hospital in St. Paul. Dowling was a truly remarkable man, despite the loss of his legs and a part of one arm in a blizzard when he was fifteen years old. In 1884, after the year at the Academy at Carleton that had been paid for by the Yellow Medicine County Board of Commissioners, he taught in the county's rural schools. In 1886 he became principal of the East Granite Falls public schools. The next year he moved to Renville as principal of the public schools there. During his three years in Renville he purchased a partial interest in its local newspaper, the *Renville Star*, and served as its co-publisher from April to November 1889, when he sold his share of it. In 1890 he stepped down as Renville's school principal and started a business selling insurance. From 1890 to 1892 he traveled throughout the Upper Midwest and neighboring Canada.

In 1892 Dowling returned to Renville, purchased the town's two newspapers, the *Star* and the *Renville Farmer*, and merged them into the *Star-Farmer*. Becoming interested in politics, he was appointed assistant clerk of the Minnesota legislature for the 1893 session. He joined the Republican Party, and in 1895 was elected secretary of the National Republican League. That same year he married Jennie Leonharda Bordewich, a young woman he had met during his year in Granite Falls. The couple moved to Chicago, as required for Dowling's work with the National Republican League.

In 1897 the Dowlings returned to Minnesota. Michael sold the *Star-Farmer* and purchased an interest in the Renville State Bank. His interest in politics remained strong. In 1897 he was appointed chief clerk of the Minnesota House of Representatives, and in 1900 he was elected a state representative; his colleagues elected him to serve as Speaker of the House. Two years later he made an unsuccessful bid for election to the United

States Senate. That year he moved his family to Olivia, where he bought a controlling interest in the Olivia State Bank and served as mayor from 1912 to 1914.[16]

Dowling was a man filled with optimism and energy. After his move to Olivia he became increasingly active as a public speaker on issues concerning disabled citizens, particularly children and veterans. He traveled overseas to conferences on the disabled as a representative of the United States government. In 1920 he made his last attempt at public office. He pursued the Republican Party nomination for governor but later withdrew his name in favor of the eventual nominee, Jacob Preus.[17]

Dowling's accomplishments, in the face of his disability, inspired many. In 1919 Dr. Nils Juel, an educator at the University of Minnesota, conceived the idea of creating a school for the crippled children of the city of Minneapolis. His suggestion was adopted by the Minneapolis Board of Education and supported by the Minnesota Rotarians. Located in south Minneapolis near the West River Road, the Michael Dowling School opened on May 3, 1920.

Following Dowling's death, the Minnesota Bankers Association and the Minnesota Editorial Association joined together to pursue the goal of building another Dowling School for crippled children. Noting the success of the Dowling school for the children of Minneapolis, the two associations wanted a school that would be open to any disabled

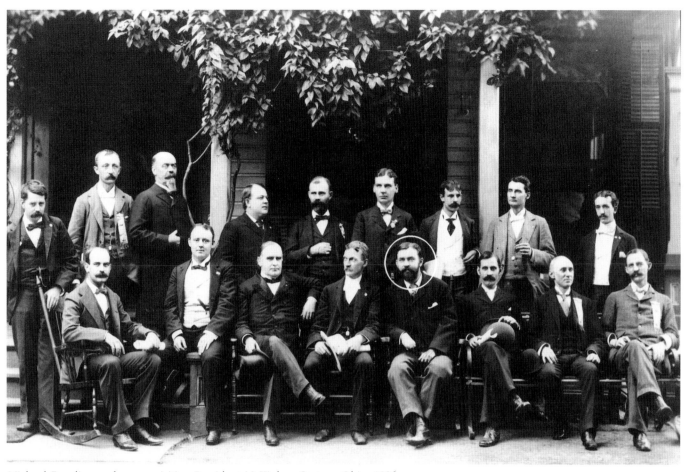

Michael Dowling and group visiting President McKinley, Canton, Ohio, 1896

child from the state of Minnesota. They began their fund drive with the slogan "Help Us to Help Them," and a goal of one hundred thousand dollars, but raised only fifty thousand dollars in the first two years. At the same time the Michael Dowling School in Minneapolis outgrew its facility, and the Minneapolis Board of Education turned to the Dowling Fund for support in building a new structure. This request, however, was not consistent with the goals of the bankers and editors, and after much discussion they decided to turn to the legislature for help in completing their own fund drive.

Perhaps mindful of Dowling's public life and service to citizens throughout the state, the legislature agreed to support the project, but decided that the school should be placed as a separate building next to the State Hospital for Indigent Crippled and Deformed Children at Lake Phalen. Chapter 297 of the Laws of 1923 gave it a name in establishing "a school for the education and training of indigent crippled and deformed children of the State of Minnesota, which shall be known as the Michael J. Dowling Memorial Hall."

The legislature appropriated fifty thousand dollars, on condition that the organizers of the Dowling fund drive provide an equal sum in cash within a year. Against that event, the legislature set aside an additional ten thousand dollars for furnishings in the new building. The entire project was placed under the State Board of Control as a part of the State Hospital for Indigent Crippled and Deformed Children.[18]

Again, Clarence Johnston designed the school, and construction started in late 1924. The building was erected just west of the hospital complex. The original landscape drawings placed its long axis in a north-south orientation, but Johnston abandoned this in favor of placing the building parallel to Ivy Avenue. The school opened on August 15, 1925, in a public ceremony attended by Jennie (Bordewich) Dowling and a large number of visitors and dignitaries. A tablet with the following inscription was placed in the building:

> The Michael J. Dowling
> Memorial Hall
>   Built and Dedicated
> by His Friends Through
> the Efforts of the Minnesota
> Editorial Association and
> Minnesota Bankers
> Association
>   That the Children Who
> Attend Here, With Imagina-
> tions Fired by the Story of This
> Man of Dauntless Spirit, May
> Achieve the Best in Life, For,
> Though Crippled in Body, He
> Was not Crippled in Mind, But
> Was a Torchbearer of Courage,
> An Inspiration of Hope, To All
> About Him.[19]

The Michael Dowling School in Minneapolis also was rebuilt. In 1923 William Henry Eustis, a millionaire, a former mayor of Minneapolis, and a man who was disabled as a child, donated land and money for a new school building and a new children's hospital at the University of Minnesota. Eustis also was instrumental in acquiring land along the East River Road, south of the University campus, which became the site of the Shriners Hospital.[20]

Jennie (Bordewich) Dowling remained involved in the affairs of people with disabilities. In 1928 she was a founder of the Society for Crippled Children and Adults. Ten years later she helped launch a camping program for the Society that was a forerunner of Camp Courage.[21]

On May 15, 1923, Dr. Arthur B. Ancker died of a heart attack in his office at City and County Hospital. He was seventy-two years old. Through his efforts, City and County Hospital was built into a high-quality facility that served the citizens of St. Paul extremely well. Shortly after his death, the hospital was renamed Ancker Hospital, and it remained at its site until 1965. That October the hospital's patients were moved to a new facility at the intersection of University Avenue and Jackson Street. The hospital was renamed St. Paul-Ramsey Hospital, retaining the connection between the city and the county, but using a new name as the hospital moved off in new directions.[22]

Judge Stephen Mahoney, the University of Minnesota regent who played such a vital role in crafting the original rules for the hospital for crippled children, died at the University of Minnesota Hospital on November 18, 1932, at the age of nearly eighty. Mahoney was the first university graduate to serve as a regent. Between 1897 and 1907, when he retired from the board of regents, Stephen Mahoney and Arthur Gillette defined the work of the hospital. We can only speculate about the direction the hospital might have taken if it had remained under the control of the regents and the supervision of Mahoney and Gillette.[23]

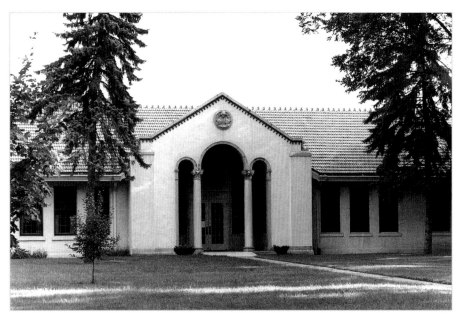

Michael J. Dowling Memorial Hall, 1975

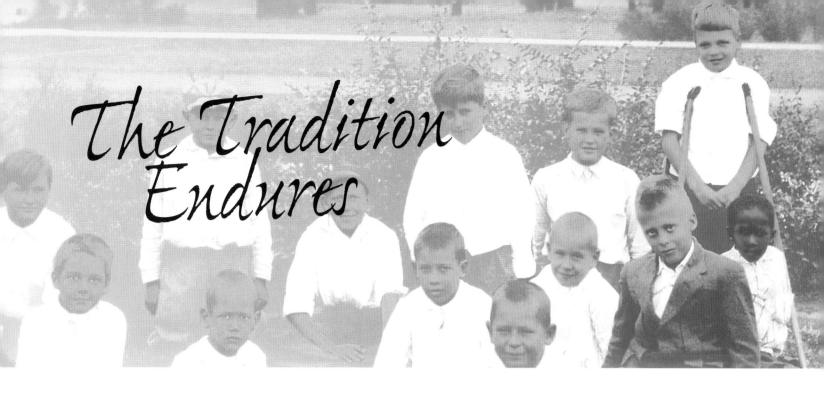

The Tradition Endures

On May 11, 1921, Elizabeth McGregor received a short letter from Downer Mullen, secretary to the State Board of Control.[1]

Dear Madam:

The Board has today appointed C. C. Chatterton, M. D., surgeon-in-chief of the State Hospital for Crippled Children, said appointment to take effect at once.

Very truly yours,
Downer Mullen, Secretary

Carl Chatterton was born on September 18, 1885, in Peterson, Iowa, a small farm community. His father, Dr. Allen Chatterton, was the town's family doctor, and Carl was drawn to medicine by his father's work. He attended medical school at Northwestern University in Chicago. At first, his interest was obstetrics. In 1910, in his final year of medical school, his class was notified that internship positions were available at City and County Hospital in St. Paul, and

interested students were told to complete a written examination.

Medical students at Northwestern were accustomed to weekly examinations. One week, soon after the notice from St. Paul arrived, an examiner failed to appear, and Chatterton and three classmates decided to fill the time by writing the examination for City and County Hospital. The papers were sent to St. Paul, and a few weeks later when Dr. Arthur Ancker came to Chicago to interview

the four students, he offered Chatterton a two-year position. The first year was to be a regular internship, working in the various departments of City and County Hospital; the second year was to be spent in the wards of the crippled children's hospital working with Arthur Gillette. Chatterton accepted the offer and arrived in St. Paul in June 1910.[2]

There are no records of Chatterton's experiences during those two years. Later, he recalled

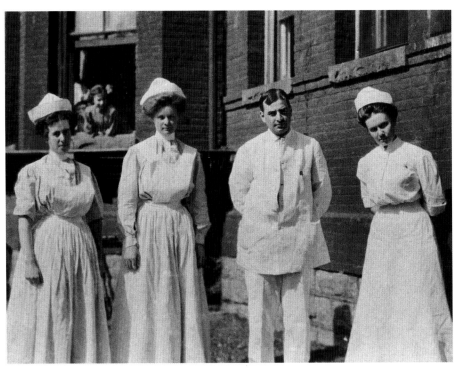

Dr. Carl Chatterton and nurses, 1911

the advice Ancker had given him during the year he worked under Dr. Gillette: "If you watch your P's and Q's you might land a job with Dr. Gillette." This proved to be prophetic; in 1912 Chatterton began work in Gillette's private office in St. Paul, and they remained partners until Gillette's death. After the hospital's move to Lake Phalen, Chatterton replaced Gillette on the list of orthopaedic surgeons printed in the annual reports of City and County Hospital.[3] Gillette actively included Chatterton in his work. The two men made a presentation to the annual meeting of the Minnesota Medical Association in 1917 that became the lead article in the first issue of the new medical journal, *Minnesota Medicine.*[4] In 1918, as Dr. Gillette's health noticeably began to fail, Chatterton was listed as associate surgeon-in-chief in

the annual report of the State Hospital for Indigent Crippled and Deformed Children. He served as surgeon-in-chief, or chief of staff, as the position later was renamed, until 1955.[5]

Chatterton was a quiet and gentle man. His work at the hospital seemed to satisfy him, and he showed little interest in national recognition. Jean Conklin, who became hospital superintendent in 1949, remembered him as "one of the nicest men I ever met. He was calm, peaceful, sympathetic . . . and a good surgeon. I don't know of a person that disliked him." But while he was a dominant figure within the hospital, he was overshadowed in the local and national medical community by Dr. Wallace Cole.[6]

Cole was born in 1888 in Fort Custer, Montana, to Hayden and Mary Cole. His father, a graduate of the United States Military Academy at West Point, was a career cavalry officer, and eventually he was stationed at Fort Snelling. Apparently this was his last post before retiring from the army, and he chose to stay in St. Paul and work in the real estate business. Wallace Cole attended undergraduate and medical school at the University of Minnesota.

In 1910 he joined Carl Chatterton and began a one-year internship at City and County Hospital, completing his work in June 1911. He next spent a year studying pathology at Johns Hopkins University in Baltimore. In 1912 Cole went to Boston, where he studied anatomy and dissection at Boston Children's Hospital and Massachusetts General Hospital.

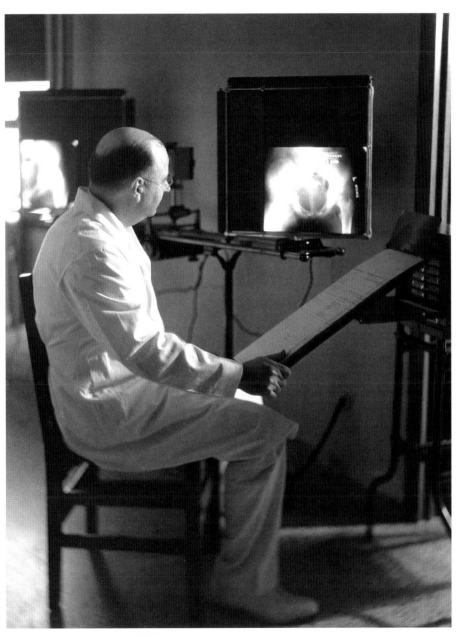

Dr. Carl Chatterton, circa 1940

The only doctor I remember is Dr. Chatterton. All of us kids use to call him "Dr. Chatterbox," and then we would all laugh because we thought that was so funny. All of us kids there seemed to like him real well. He just talked with us kids, and maybe teased, and was always kind of a jolly man. He was a happy, friendly, guy.

Elizabeth (Gawreluk) Wilson
1993

He was a big teddy bear. I can remember his bald head.

Jean (Schilling) Legried
1993

He was old and kind and gentle.

Rosemary (Ackermann) Johnson
1993

From Boston, Cole traveled to Liverpool, England, where in 1913 he spent several months working with Robert Jones. At that time Jones was at the forefront in the emergence in Great Britain of orthopaedics as a medical specialty.[7]

Cole's travels also took him to Europe, but by 1914 he had returned to St. Paul. He was a member of the Ramsey County Medical Society, and his name, along with Carl Chatterton's, was listed in the 1914 Annual Report of City and County Hospital. He opened an office in the Lowry Medical Arts Building and joined the staff of the State Hospital for Indigent Crippled and Deformed Children.[8]

Cole quickly became active in other medical groups in the Twin Cities. He published an article in the *The St. Paul Medical Journal* in 1915, and joined a group of young specialists who wrote a section for the journal titled "Progress in Medicine." His first orthopaedic contribution was a review of an article by Robert Jones on derangements of the knee, previously published in the well-known journal *Surgery, Gynecology, and Obstetrics.*[9] In 1915 the Central States Orthopedic Society held its fifth annual meeting in Minnesota. The first day of the meeting was hosted by Dr. Gillette at the hospital at Lake Phalen. He gave a tour, presented some cases, then put his two young colleagues in the limelight for the rest of the morning. Dr. Chatterton presented cases of infection and one unusual case of an aneurysm that formed after surgery to bone graft a fracture that would not heal. Dr. Cole presented six cases that showed the diversity of problems seen at the hospital at that time. These included a child with brittle bones, another with tuberculosis of the hip, a teenager who had been paralyzed after being born in a breech position, and three cases of surgical techniques to correct wrist weakness, knee contracture, and hip dislocation due to polio.[10]

Hayden Cole's military career is certain to have left an impression on his son. After his return to St. Paul, Dr. Cole joined the Minnesota National Guard, but not its medical corps; he was a field artillery officer. In 1916 President Woodrow Wilson activated the National Guard as part of the United States military effort to capture Pancho Villa in northern Mexico. Cole's unit, the First Minnesota Field Artillery, was sent to a border area near Columbus, New Mexico. Cole remained there for nine months as commander of Battery A. In March 1917 he returned to St. Paul, where he was commissioned a captain in the United States Army medical corps. A month later the United States entered the war in Europe.[11]

The American orthopaedic community had been preparing for the war since 1914. According to Leonard Peltier, a prominent orthopaedic surgeon and historian, American volunteer orthopaedic surgeons serving in France had convinced local planners that the wounded needed specialized orthopaedic care. A list of young orthopaedic surgeons was drawn

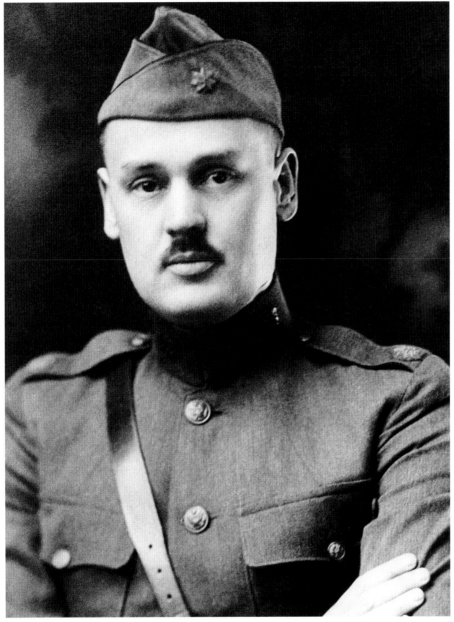

Dr. Wallace Cole, circa 1916

Oh, I liked him! He always had a little joke or something to tell you. He was a very pleasant man.

**Sharon (Osborn) Johnson
about Dr. Cole, 1993**

When I first met him, I was just awestruck. He was very nice. He was a distinguished looking man, and he was a very, very nice person. He had a very nice personality.

**Marlene Gardner
about Dr. Cole, 1993**

up by Joel Goldthwait, an orthopaedic surgeon from Boston who was chairman of committees on war preparedness that had been established by the American Orthopaedic Association and the orthopaedic section of the American Medical Association. Goldthwait knew Arthur Gillette well. Both had been president of the American Orthopaedic Association (Gillette in 1900, Goldthwait in 1907), and in December 1907, during Gillette's term as president of the Minnesota Academy of Medicine, Goldthwait had been invited to Minnesota to deliver a talk on rheumatic joint conditions. This connection may have brought Cole to Boston for his year of study.[12]

When America entered the

war, the British asked for twenty orthopaedic surgeons to work with Robert Jones. Wallace Cole was one of the men Joel Goldthwait selected. The group sailed from New York and arrived in Liverpool on May 28, 1917. The plan was for the members of the group, later referred to as the Goldthwait Unit, to be sent to military orthopaedic hospitals in Britain. After they had gained experience treating war injuries, and after the American Expeditionary Force entered combat, they would be transferred to military hospitals in France. Cole was assigned to the Alder Hey Military Hospital outside Liverpool, a facility Jones had personally organized. Later, Cole was sent to Bordeaux, France, where he and J. C. Graves supervised an orthopaedic hospital containing twenty thousand beds. His last post was a military hospital near Oxford, England. After the armistice of November 11, 1918, work in the military hospitals quickly dwindled, and Dr. Cole returned to St. Paul the following May. He resumed his practice and his work at the State Hospital for Indigent Crippled and Deformed Children. As he wrote many years later: "The old arrangements were resumed. Dr. Chatterton was assigned the boys, and I was assigned the girls."[13]

As Peltier points out, the members of the Goldthwait Unit went on to dominate American orthopaedics for the next thirty years. Beginning in 1921, Dr. Cole served as secretary of the Clinical Orthopaedic Society for two years. He then was vice president for a

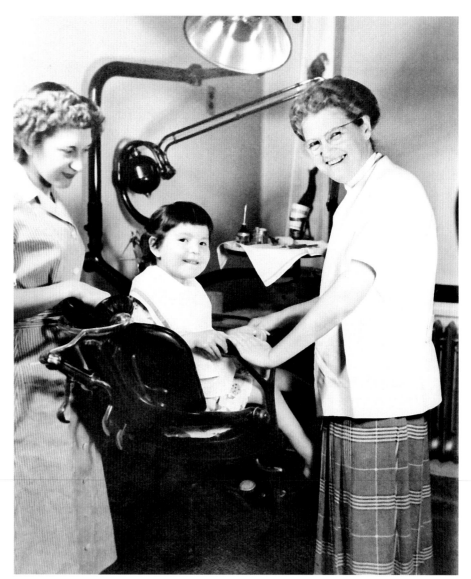

Dr. Grace Jones, circa 1950

year before becoming president. His first scholarly publication after the war surely was a reflection of his experiences with Robert Jones and the war. Titled "The Use of the Thomas Knee Splint for the Routine Treatment of Fracture of the Shaft of the Femur," it was published in *Minnesota Medicine* in 1920. The Thomas Splint, brought to the war effort by Jones, had resulted in a dramatic reduction in deaths caused by fractures of the femur in which the bone fragments

had ruptured through the muscle and skin of the thigh. In 1916 British Army statistics showed that 80 percent of soldiers with such an injury died. By 1917, through the use of the splint, this had been reduced to 15.6 percent. It was one of several reasons that Robert Jones received a knighthood.[14]

After Dr. Chatterton was named the hospital's surgeon-in-chief, Dr. Cole was made associate surgeon-in-chief. The two men continued in these roles for more than thirty years. In 1923 the Twin Cities Unit of the Shriners Hospital for Crippled Children was opened, and Dr. Cole was appointed chief surgeon, a position he held until 1953. In 1928 he was elected president of the Ramsey County Medical Society. In 1929 Owen Wangensteen, chairman of the department of surgery, named him professor of orthopaedics and chairman of the division of orthopaedic surgery at the University of Minnesota, a post Dr. Gillette had once held.[15]

Almost everyone who met Wallace Cole noticed his quiet, reserved manner, his upright posture, his timeliness, and his attention to detail. Jean Conklin described him as "a highly intelligent man. He never pushed himself [on others]. He let people come and seek him." He also was very consistent. Conklin described his preferences in clothing and cars: "He was a perfect gentleman. He was beautifully dressed all the time, but you would never guess it was a new suit because it was in the same material and same style as the old one. The same with his cars. He drove Jaguars, but he got them so they looked alike. I remember he was getting a new car and he told the girls that when he came the next Thursday he'd have a new car. They were all anxiously looking out the windows when he drove up and got out. He came down to the ward and said, 'Well, did you see the new car?' They said, 'It looks just like the old one!' And it did."

Dr. Cole also was a gifted teacher. The house doctors, or residents, told Jean Conklin how much his teaching meant to them: "The residents used to sit spellbound when he'd open up and really talk. . . . They said they learned more in those sessions than they did in anything else."[16]

In 1924 Grace Jones, a remarkable young woman, arrived at the hospital to serve as its dentist for the next forty-five years. Grace was born in Cleveland, Minnesota, on August 28, 1900. She was one of three children. Her father was a cashier in a bank in a village near Bemidji. He died of tuberculosis when Grace was twelve years old, and to support her family, Grace's mother took in boarders. Grace attended high school in Bemidji, and then worked in a railroad machine shop for a year and a half during World War I.

After the war Grace planned to attend the state teacher's college at St. Cloud and become a grade school teacher, but her older brother had gone to dental school in Chicago, loved his work, and strongly encouraged Grace to consider dentistry. Responding to his enthusiasm and promise of support, she applied for a position in the dental college at the University of Minnesota. Despite the competition for dental school openings, the entrance committee was impressed by her work during the war. She was the only woman in her class and younger than her classmates, many of whom had served in the wartime military. None of this caused her any problems. As she described it, "The boys treated me just like their kid

I was going to go to St. Cloud and take a two year grade school teaching degree but my brother was eight years older than I was and he was already out and he was a dentist because he fell in love with dentistry after he took his business course. He went to Chicago. He said, "I'll help you if you take dentistry." Well, anything to get an education. I really wasn't particular about it. It worked out very wonderful.

**Dr. Grace Jones
1994**

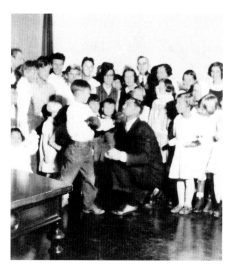

Boxer Jack Dempsey visits, 1931

sister." She was twenty-three years old when she graduated.

Grace worked with her brother for six months, then applied for the job at the hospital at Phalen Park. She worked part-time, three days a week. The dental facilities she found there were very basic, to say the least: "My [first] office was a bay window in the switchboard room. We had no running water, a chair, but no suction. So the next year they built an addition. . . . I had a tiny room, but they did not realize that I had to bring beds into the room. We could just squeeze the beds in. I had a new chair that went way down to the floor so we could push the beds on top. It overlooked the formal gardens. . . . I kept my supplies and things on a shelf in the cast room."

A lot of the children in the hospital needed dental work, and Grace worked hard: "Those kids came from all over the state. They came by bus and train and streetcar. [The hospital] was very, very, busy and full. . . . The kids came in for lots of things, not just orthopaedics. . . . They hadn't had a permanent dentist for a couple of years. So, I had every kid in the place to look at. In those days there were a lot of cavities. That's one thing about the job. It got easier and easier as I worked there because we had flouride in the water, and we had flouride in the toothpaste. But, at first, no."

Many of the children had never seen a dentist. She remembered that "everybody had dental work that needed to be done. You see, in those days they did not think that it was necessary to fill the baby teeth. They forgot that they hold the space for the ones that are coming when they are eight and ten years old. And, behind them come the six-year molars. . . . Lots of kids never had a toothbrush, and those that did just brushed on Saturday night when they took a bath. There was no dental hygiene taught in school."

In fact, the work was overwhelming. In addition to the dozens and dozens of children with cavities, Grace was confronted by many, many children who had developed abscesses under their teeth. They needed their teeth removed or their abscesses drained. Dr. Chatterton helped by obtaining the services of an oral surgeon, who came once a month and did his work in the operating room while the children were under anesthesia.

By her account, Grace performed approximately fifty thousand dental procedures during her years at the hospital. Many children saw her more than once. Her days developed a routine. Children from the outpatient department were seen in the morning, those from the wards in the afternoon. Grace kept a list of children who needed dental work. Monica Reilly, her long-time dental assistant, was sent to the wards to "find whatever kid was available. It didn't make any difference to me." The children dreaded a trip to the dental office. Grace never used numbing medicine. Instead, "I just talked to them. I cleaned their teeth first. We had no trouble. Well, I can't say no trouble. . . . I talked to them, and Monica talked to them and got their attention."

Occasionally one of the children would challenge her: "Boys talked constantly. Girls in that day and age were a little on the shy side. . . . There was the boy that came in and said, 'I am going to let you look at my teeth. Did you go someplace to learn how?' I told him that I had gone to high school and four years of college and then I told him that I had to take a state examination. He then asked if I had passed."

Grace was impressed by all the people who worked as volunteers. "There was a lady that taught vocal lessons. I saw her in June, and I said, 'Why don't you take a vacation?' She told me that she was working with two girls, ages fourteen and fifteen. They were from small towns. She said, 'They have as nice a voice as I have ever heard. I want to teach them all that I can before they go home, and I want to get through to them that they are just as good

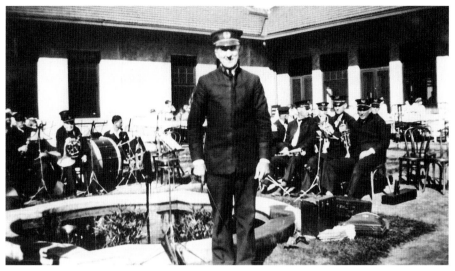

Bandleader with his band, circa 1930

as anybody in their town, and that they should sing every chance they could get.' I thought that was dedication. That was free, volunteer work."

Grace remembered "the volunteer that was teaching southern songs to the kids in the ward, from six to twelve years old. She had a map of the South, and she was showing them where Kentucky was, and what they grew in Kentucky, and the homes.

Those were the things that impressed me the most, the education that everybody was trying to teach those kids. When they got out, they knew something."[17]

Sometimes the regular teachers had to scramble: "They had five teachers, regular grade school and high school teachers. Once they forgot to hire one that could teach physics, and this boy had to pass his physics examination to graduate in June. So the Latin teacher taught him. She studied under the midnight oil, and once in a while she would have to go to the high school on the way home and have the physics teacher help her."[18]

The children received visits from many celebrities. They included the Queen of Norway, boxer Jack Dempsey, the Lone Ranger, Sky King, Gene Autry and the Sons of the Pioneers, and, later, Harmon Killebrew of the Minnesota Twins. Grace Jones remembered the visit of another baseball player. One afternoon she was in one of the

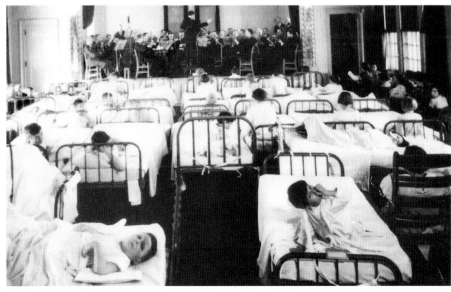

Kids in the auditorium to hear an orchestra, circa 1930

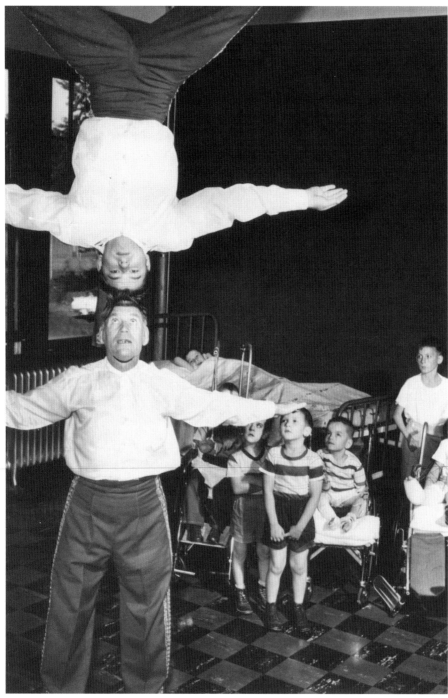

Circus acrobats, circa 1930

bed if Babe sat on it."[19]

The number of applications for care always exceeded the capacity of the hospital. As polio became more common, the waiting list for admission grew, often to more than two hundred names. Dr. Chatterton recruited more physicians and developed a medical staff that included specialists in every major medical field. In 1924 Drs. A. E. Flagstad and W. H. Von der Weyer joined the staff as attending orthopaedic surgeons; they were followed by George Williamson (1928), John Moe (1934), S. W. Shimonek (1936), Meyer Goldner (1940), Harry Hall (1948), Donovan McCain (1948), and John Beer, Frank Babb, Lester Carlander, and Richard Johnson in the early 1950s. The physicians continued to donate their services, but Chatterton found it hard to recruit the help he needed. In 1930 he appealed to the board of control for permission to include stipends for physicians in the hospital's annual budget. This was denied until 1938, when physicians were granted $50 a month to cover automobile expenses. By 1942, when the hospital was no longer supervised by the board of control, total physician compensation reached $7,000.[20]

With so many children waiting for admission, the hospital was openly supportive of the new Shriners Hospital in Minneapolis. There seemed to be more than enough children to keep both hospitals busy. As Miss McGregor observed: "There is [a] need for more hospitals, and

wards and "all of a sudden the whole ward said 'Hi, Babe!' The biggest guy I ever saw had come in. It was Babe Ruth. Boy! They had four boys who were in traction, and when he saw this those tears rolled down

this great big guy. He was getting ready to sit down when the nurse came back with a big metal chair. He was going to sit down on the edge of the bed, and we held our breath. All of us knew that there would be no

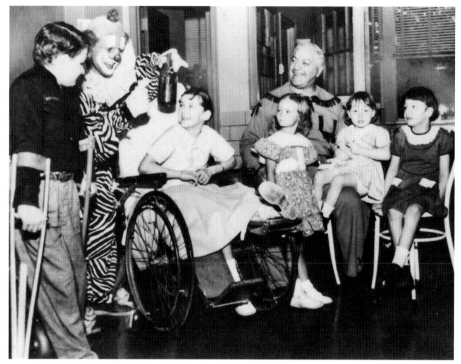

Clarabelle and Buffalo Bob entertaining girls, circa 1931

anyone wishing to start such a movement, or who will do anything to interest the public in caring for the crippled children will have the most hearty support of all those in the work." Miss McGregor and Dr. Cole were consulted when the Shriners Hospital was being designed, and after it opened, the two hospitals worked together closely. It was common for them to share their waiting lists in order to avoid duplication of services.[21]

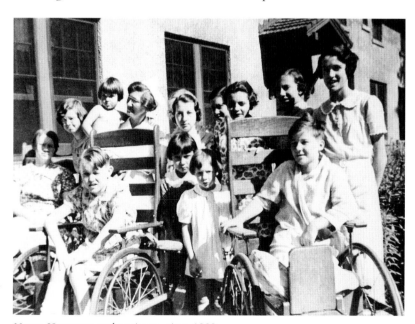

Nurse Hostetter and patients, circa 1930

After Congress passed the National Security Act in 1936, federal dollars began to flow into Minnesota for the care of children with disabilities. The legislature created a Department of Social Security, with a Division of Public Institutions, and with that, the State Board of Control was disbanded. The hospital remained under the Public Institutions division until the legislature reorganized the Department of Social Security and created a Department of Public Welfare. Federal money allowed the state to fund some health care in communities closer to a child's home. It also allowed the state to expand the small network of field clinics the hospital had established in the 1920s. The clinics expanded rapidly, and they were given four tasks by the state. They were asked to follow-up established patients, find more children with disabilities, provide preventive health education, and provide consultative services for community physicians.[22]

Through all these years Elizabeth McGregor continued to run the hospital with a firm hand. In 1933 she was among the one hundred men and thirteen women who founded the American College of Hospital Administrators. The hospital continued to be examined by the American College of Surgeons and to maintain its Class A rating. It was not a small enterprise. The hospital's budget grew steadily. Its biennial budget for 1919–20 was $228,500; for 1929–30 it was $372,350; for 1939–40, $485,000; for 1949–50 it reached $1,383,618. Through the eyes of a child, Miss McGregor seemed a tough taskmaster. She was, but the hospital needed supervision. Those who worked with her knew that and respected her and her work.

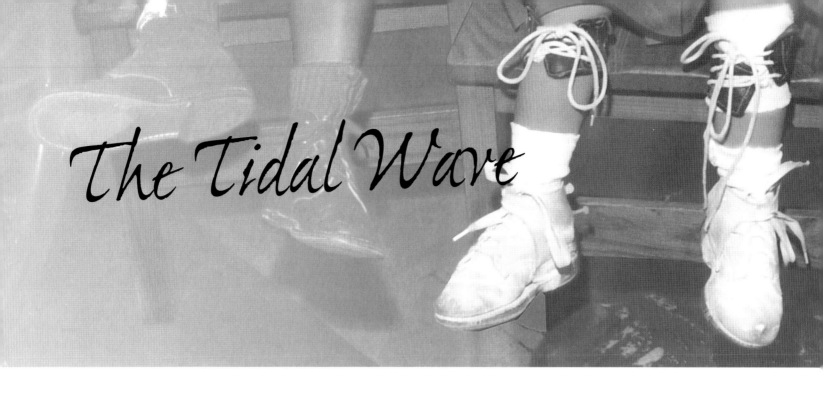

The Tidal Wave

It is difficult to explain the fear of polio to anyone born in the closing decades of the twentieth century. Polio came without warning, usually striking children and teenagers. It paid no attention to the skin color, gender, or social standing of its victims. It often came in waves, creating panic and overwhelming local hospitals. In 1952, at its peak, this plague struck more than fifty-two thousand people in the United States. Polio was every parent's nightmare.

"Polio" is the shortened version of the proper medical term, anterior poliomyelitis. When polio struck, the usual outcome was weakness of muscles, which varied from one person to the next. Some had little or no permanent weakness; others were left paralyzed, sometimes to the extent that they could breath only with a mechanical ventilator, or "iron lung." The word poliomyelitis is derived from two Greek words: polios, meaning "gray," and myelos, meaning "matter," words referring to a specific part of the brain and spinal cord. When viewed with the naked eye, groups of nerve cells which specialize in sending impulses to muscle cells have a darker, or grayer, appearance than other parts of the nervous system. Within the spinal cord, these cells are clustered in the front half of the cord, hence the term anterior poliomyelitis. A particular group of viruses, first described in 1908 in Vienna by Drs. Karl Landsteiner and Erwin Popper, are able to infect and damage these nerve cells, robbing their ability to activate muscle cells. Weakness or paralysis is the result.[1]

Polio was not new. People with polio deformities were pictured in drawings from ancient Egypt, and medical texts from the Middle Ages described the weakness it caused. What was new were the virulent epidemics of severe, disabling polio. During the height of the polio epidemic years in North America, the medical director of the Children's Hospital in Cairo, Egypt, told Dr. John Paul, a leading American polio researcher that "Poliomyelitis

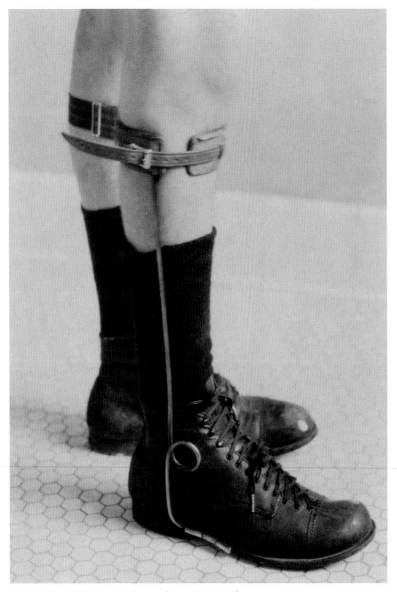

Spring-loaded short leg brace for polio, 1926

they were affected by the virus, they were less sick. Inevitably, children living under better sanitary conditions grew up with less exposure to the virus. They were more susceptible to infection, and the results often were devastating. Initially, researchers believed the virus was inhaled, perhaps passing into the olfactory nerves, which were specialized for smell, and from there directly to the brain. This theory led to treatments designed to stop the spread of the disease during epidemics. Compounds of picric acid or zinc sulfate were sprayed into the noses of children. This proved useless because the theory was wrong. Several researchers discovered large quantities of the polio virus in human feces. The place of entry for the virus was not the nose, it was the bowel.[2]

The stories of four young people who were patients at Gillette State Hospital for Crippled Children illustrate how quickly polio could develop, and how serious the illness could be.

Burton Aarness was a healthy nineteen-year-old in the fall of 1921. He was working in the harvest fields near Thief River Falls when he became ill.

> We had an excellent binder for cutting grain, but this day, with fair weather, a level field, and not too heavy grain, one thing went wrong after another. It was pesky. Only one round was made on what I estimate to be a forty acre field, in the forenoon. At noon the horses were

is not rare in Egypt. It is never epidemic, always sporadic. . . . The cases as a rule are mild, involving only one limb, rarely a fatality." That was not the western European and North American experience. There, polio represented a cruel paradox. The discovery of microbes such as bacteria and the viruses in the nineteenth century was followed by improved public sanitation and cleaner food and water.

As a result, public health improved, and diseases such as tuberculosis began to fade. But not polio. Instead of disappearing, it exploded in epidemic waves.

Public health measures did not cause polio, however; they simply made people more susceptible to the virus. Earlier, the viruses that caused polio had been more common in the population. Children developed a natural immunity at an early age, and if unhitched and watered and fed. On the way going to the house my foot would sometimes miss and I would nearly fall to the ground. I must have had a small meal and felt so miserable that no grain cutting was attempted in the afternoon. Towards evening the folks came home. I was so indescribably miserable. I could not remain in bed, and it was just as bad to be up. This continued through the night and in the morning my legs would not function. Dr. Atkins . . . was called and he drove out the fourteen miles and immediately diagnosed poliomyelitis. For me it was the most painful time. After not sleeping for two weeks because of the pain, medication for sleep was given. The usual sleeping potions were administered, I took them, and I stayed awake. Finally, chloroform was administered orally, one drop, then two and three. Still no sleep. Then a half teaspoonful. This caused the worst wrenching of my heart, causing me to scream. However, after that I slept for three hours. After three weeks of pain I began feeling better, I was able to be up and about. I had lost twenty pounds.

Burton was admitted to the hospital in 1922 and stayed seven months. He was admitted again in 1928 and stayed six weeks.[3]

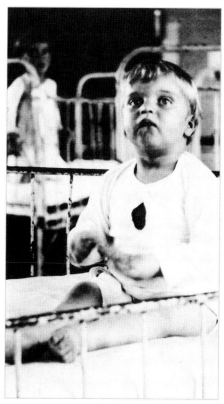

Polio patient Ernest Charley Johnson, 1922

Clara (Janzen) Trout was fourteen years old in 1931. She and her family were members of a Mennonite community near Mountain Lake.

I had just turned fourteen. It was in July. We were in church that Sunday, but church was outside because of the polio epidemic. That is the Sunday I started getting headaches. By Monday my headaches were so severe that walking even hurt. By Tuesday I was in bed and really sick. We did not know what it was. My mother had a cousin who was an osteopath and, well, we thought that maybe with the right eating and all of that I would get better, but

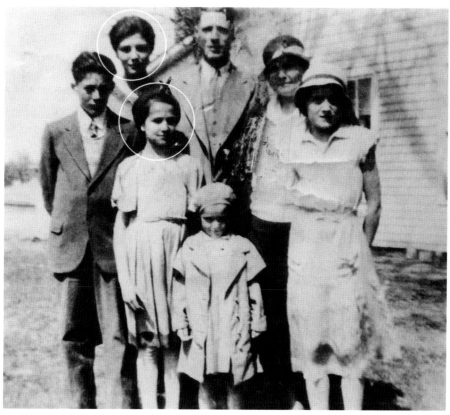

Marie and Marjorie Bassett and her family on their Blue Earth farm, 1931

I didn't. So the doctor, Dr. Piper, was called in. By that time we knew what it was because I could not move some of my parts. It was my left leg especially, and my right leg, too. Actually, Dr. Piper did not do that much for me. Well, what could he do? I don't think that he knew. He just kept me in bed. He told us to force fluid, and kind of a little pill that they gave me, too. I don't know what it was, but I think it was to bring the fever down. It was quite a long siege.

Clara was admitted to the hospital two months later and stayed for nine months.[4]

In 1930 Marjorie (Bassett) Simon was a happy eight-year-old, living with her family on a farm near Blue Earth.

It was the fall of 1930 that the lives of two children of the Bassett family were to be changed for all their years to come. That fall the Blue Earth school had opened and had been in session for a few weeks. I was happily anticipating being a second-grader. One day, shortly after the start of school, I came home feeling quite ill. My mom kept me at home since I wasn't getting any better. Shortly after my getting sick my older sister, Marie, who was a freshman in high school, began not feeling well. After she had fallen down the steps at

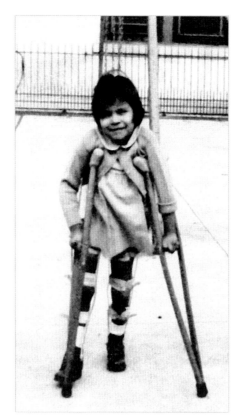

Young polio patient wearing long leg braces, 1949

school a couple of times, my parents decided to see the one doctor in our small town to find out what ailed the two of us. He rather casually stated that we had arthritis and would recover with rest at home. I'm sure it seemed strange to my parents for the two of us to have a disease attributed mostly to the elderly, but they seemed to accept it. Our home rest went on for a few weeks with no recovery in sight when a relative in St. Paul found out about our problem and suggested that our parents take Marie and me to Gillette Hospital for a check-up. . . . Of course, they immediately diagnosed our illness as polio.

Marjorie had two short stays in the hospital, for a month in 1931 and two months in 1937.[5]

Karen (Oberg) Valerius grew up in St. Paul as one of three children. Her father was a fireman, and would become St. Paul's fire chief.

In the summer of 1945, when I was five years old, my mother took me and my girlfriend to the grocery store. We exchanged lollipops halfway home. Later that day I began to feel ill. My little brother, who was a year old, crawled up on the couch with me. I told him to get down or I would give him my germs, and I blew on him. The next morning I was having difficulty talking and swallowing. Meningitis was suspected, but paralysis spread and polio was diagnosed by Dr. Gilbert Wenzel. Fortunately, neither my friend nor my brother got polio.[6]

The ability of the polio virus to strike at will, without regard for the status of its victim, became clear in the case of Franklin Delano Roosevelt, who was an emerging political force when he became ill in August 1921. He had been the Democratic vice presidential nominee in 1920, and before that was an assistant secretary of the Navy. He was young, forty years old, charismatic, and energetic. More than fifty years after his death, it is tempting to portray his physical and political recovery in grand

and triumphant terms. In fact, his recovery was slow, difficult, and incomplete. Although he returned to public life, became governor of New York, and later president of the United States, as well as an inspiration for polio victims everywhere, he did not willingly display his disability. To the public, he wished to appear whole.

Roosevelt became the focus of a national effort to treat and eradicate polio. The effort began with his purchase of a spa built over natural thermal springs in Warm Springs, Georgia. There he built a rehabilitation center for polio victims and created the Warm Springs Foundation to attract donations to aid financially needy victims. After his election to the presidency, a series of national President's Birthday Balls were organized to raise money for the foundation. Eventually the proceeds from the balls were divided between local charities and research grants to scientists studying the polio virus. Finally, in 1937, the National Foundation for Infantile Paralysis (NFIP) was formed to, as Roosevelt described it, "lead, direct, and unify the fight on every phase of this sickness."

The NFIP was, in part, a response to scandal. In 1935 the rush to produce results in the war on polio resulted in the use of two new, partially tested, vaccines. Drs. William Park and Maurice Brodie of the New York Health Department laboratories and Dr. John Kolmer of Temple University in Philadelphia administered their vaccines to nine thousand and twelve thousand children, respectively. Within months, polio developed among those immunized, and some children died. Park and Brodie had received funding from the Presidential Birthday Balls Commission (PBBC). The disaster damaged the PBBC's credibility and donations dropped off. The NFIP was an effort to separate Roosevelt from the fight against polio and also attract

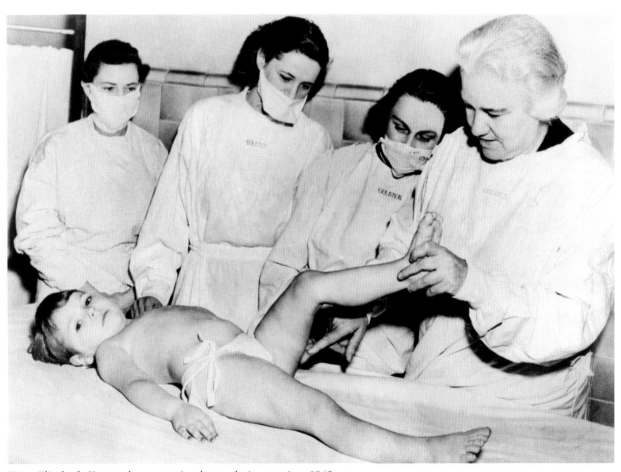

Sister Elizabeth Kenny demonstrating her techniques, circa 1942

more rigorous scientific minds. The move was to bear fruit in the 1950s in the development of two successful vaccines.[7]

In the early twentieth century the prevailing American medical authority for the treatment of poliomyelitis was Dr. Robert Lovett, an orthopaedic surgeon in Boston and one of Roosevelt's physicians. In 1916 he published a textbook entitled *The Treatment of Infantile Paralysis.* In it he divided treatment into three phases: acute, convalescent, and chronic. In the acute phase, which he described as lasting up to three months after onset of the illness, he advocated rest. He thought movement and therapy might damage fragile muscle tissue. Splints were used to position limbs and rest the joints. In the convalescent phase, which he considered to last up to two years after the appearance of paralysis, Lovett prescribed activity. Patients were to get up, their limbs were to be moved, and weight-bearing was encouraged. Treatment of deformities by surgical means was reserved for the chronic phase, considered to be more than two years after the onset of the illness. For thirty years, rest and splinting with braces or casts were the foundation of treatment for polio. In 1940 everything changed when Sister Elizabeth Kenny came to the United States from Australia.[8]

Elizabeth Kenny was nearly sixty years old when she arrived in San Francisco with her adopted daughter Mary. Relatively unknown then, she would become within a decade a larger-than-life figure, one of the best-known and most popular people in the United States. She had learned basic nursing skills as a bush nurse in the outback of Queensland. Her first encounter with polio, a story now shrouded in legend, came in 1911. She was called to a remote settlement where she found a severely weakened, miserable two-year-old boy. She sent a telegram to her adviser, Dr. Aeneas McDonnell, who responded with the diagnosis of poliomyelitis, and the advice that little useful could be done. Kenny prayed for guidance, then tried a series of remedies in the hope of comforting her small patient. Finally, she found something that brought relief and allowed him to sleep. She cut a heavy woolen blanket into strips, dipped the strips in boiling water, wrung them out, and then wrapped them around his limbs. As soon as the pain subsided, she moved the boy's arms and legs and encouraged him to move them on his own. He made a good recovery, and Kenny used the same method on other children in her district. She had developed the basic elements of the treatment that would make her famous.

During World War I, Kenny worked on troop ships carrying wounded Australian soldiers home, and she earned the title of "Sister," which was given to nurses in the British Commonwealth. Although she never had received any formal training as a nurse, she resumed treating polio victims in Australia in the 1930s. She met with stiff resistance from the medical establishment, but apparently her treatments were successful, and in 1935 the Queensland government formed a commission to study her results. The commission eventually condemned her methods as dangerous, but by that time Sister Kenny had left for England. A committee there was less negative, its members deeming Kenny's treatment "harmless but of unproved benefit." After her return to Australia, Kenny's supporters in the medical community convinced the Queensland government to finance a trip to the United States.

Elizabeth and Mary Kenny traveled first to New York City, where they met Basil O'Connor, director of the National Foundation for Infantile Paralysis but received no support. They traveled next to Chicago, where she met Dr. Morris Fishbein, editor of *The Journal of the American Medical Association.* He also was skeptical but sent them to the Mayo Clinic in Rochester, where they met Dr. Melvin Henderson, chairman of the orthopaedic department. Dr. Henderson was interested in Sister Kenny's ideas, but the Mayo Clinic had few patients with polio. Henderson sent the Kennys on to Minneapolis and St. Paul, and to his friend, Dr. Wallace Cole. Henderson knew that Cole, through his work at Gillette State Hospital, the Shriners Hospital, and the

University of Minnesota, had numerous polio patients, and that Cole was unhappy with the current treatment of the disease. He also knew that Cole, beneath his quiet, stern demeanor, was fair and open to new ideas.[9]

The day after Sister Kenny arrived, Cole took her to Gillette State Hospital to examine some of the children with polio. Several of those remember her visit. Bonita (Derby) Melzer

from International Falls was eleven years old at the time.

She came to the hospital and worked on me twice. What I remember was a large lady in a dark blue uniform. She had beautiful white hair, if I can remember right. She wore a necklace . . . of shiny beads that you used to see years ago. Anyway, she took those off and handed them

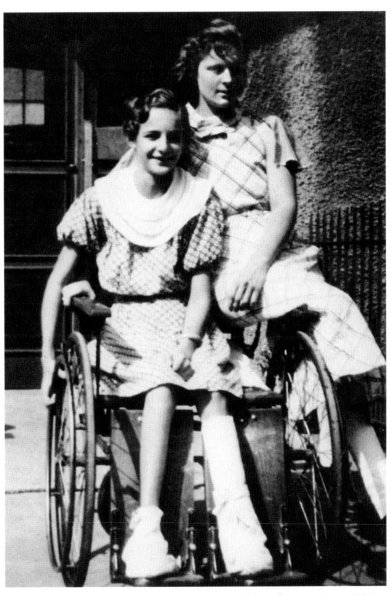

Two Gillette State Hospital patients, Norma Fricke and Mary Lieser, 1932

to me. At that time I could not do anything with my leg. . . . She would have me look at those beads and while I would look at them she would say, "Now concentrate on moving this toe," and pretty soon it would move just a little, which it never had before. I only got to have her work on me twice, but they had people just standing around. Well, we were like guinea pigs, I guess. Everybody was watching her every movement. . . . I can remember that she seemed to be a very patient person, and everybody was in awe.[10]

Elizabeth Cantwell of St. Paul was nine years old when she met Sister Kenny.

I was so impressed with her because she was so big. My mother was very concerned that I shouldn't do many activities, and [Sister Kenny] said, "She can do anything that she wants to do, and she always will do anything she wants to do." There was a real aura about it. It's real hard to explain. You know, your little withered legs, and she put this powerful hand on them and says, "Move. Tell it to move." It's like a miracle. She dressed very strangely, too. She dressed in all black and wore black oxford shoes with black socks and . . . she wore a big black hat, a big, big hat. You did not see a woman dressed in

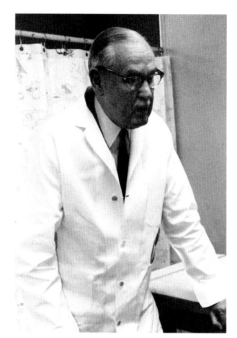

Dr. Wallace Cole, circa 1970

black in a hospital. . . . I mean, she came down the hall and, boy, it was like a parade behind her.[11]

Kenny promptly introduced her hot packs. Beverly (Lyttle) Allstopp, a ten-year-old girl from St. Paul, was one of the first children to experience this treatment.

The doctors came in a cluster. They kind of stood in awe of her. Several of us had the Sister Kenny treatment. The Maytag washing machine went down the middle of the ward with hot water in it and the wool flannels wrung out with the wringer. Then they put some rubberized material over that, and pinned the whole thing in there so that it would hold the heat. . . . They did not keep it up too well because it would get

wet, so they were not trying all that hard.[12]

Bonita (Derby) Melzer had hot packs for several months.

I remember the nurses coming with what looked like an old fashioned tub with a wringer on it. They would use wool, and they had forceps that they would pick this out of the water with, and run it through the wringer, then wrap it in a towel, and run to your back, or legs, and wrap it around real quick.[13]

Dr. Cole was impressed with Sister Kenny's first visit. He introduced her to some of his colleagues, including Dr. George Williamson, a St. Paul orthopaedic surgeon; Dr. Miland E. Knapp, a specialist in physical medicine at the University of Minnesota; and Dr. John Pohl, a Minneapolis orthopaedic surgeon. Over the next week, Sister Kenny was invited to examine polio patients at several other hospitals. Cole and Williamson were sufficiently impressed with her results that they took several children out of their casts and splints and began to treat them with her methods. Most physicians remained skeptical. It took a single, dramatic, encounter to overcome their doubts. Henry Haverstock, Jr., was one of John Pohl's patients and the son of a Minneapolis attorney. He was eighteen and had been severely paralyzed by polio in 1939. He had been to Warm Springs for treatment with little success. He was bedridden and could not even sit. Sister Kenny reversed all the treatment Henry had been given, and within a year he was able to walk with crutches. This turnabout made Pohl a convert to Sister Kenny's methods.[14]

Her ideas, however, were not easy to understand, and she did not make things easy for the medical profession or for herself. She had little sense of diplomacy, was often blunt, and even openly rude. Her lectures were boring and her explanations of scientific principles were impossible to follow. She described the weakness of polio as being the result of spasm, mental alienation, and incoordination. Of these, she thought spasm was the most important. With polio there was painful tightening and shortening of the affected muscles, which pulled against the opposing muscles and created a deformity. She also believed that the brain lost contact with the opposing muscles in a sort of mental alienation that made the weakness seem worse than it actually was. This, in turn, resulted in poorly coordinated muscle activity. Kenny believed that rest and casts caused muscles to become atrophied and fibrotic, and joints to become stiff. The sooner the pain was relieved, and the sooner the limb was moved and the muscles were put to work, the better the recovery of the child.[15]

Cole, with the help of Dr. Harold Diehl, dean of the University of Minnesota Medical School, appealed to Basil O'Connor for funds to allow Sister Kenny to stay in the Twin Cities. Cole, Knapp, and Pohl agreed that some sort of supervised trial of the Kenny method was needed to determine if its results were any different from those of standard

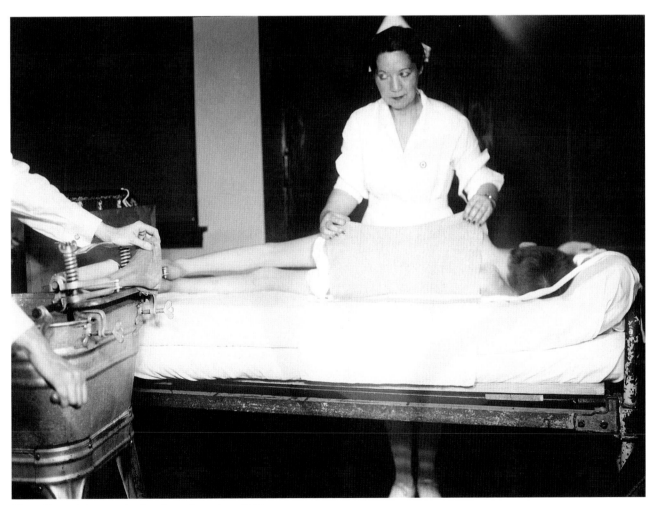

Sister Kenny's hot packs for the spine, circa 1945

95

treatment. The trial was held at Minneapolis General Hospital, where many polio victims were taken when they first became sick. In 1940 Elizabeth and Mary Kenny treated twenty-six people who either had acute polio or were in the early stages of recovery. Cole and Knapp evaluated the results and published their findings in *The Journal of the America Medical Association.*

> We think it is possible and appropriate to state definitely that these patients with acute infantile paralysis are much more comfortable and cheerful . . . than are those cases who are immobilized, and we have seen absolutely no contractures . . . following this treatment. Even the most severely paralyzed patient has passively full range of motion in all his joints. . . . We believe that the paralysis is less severe than would be expected in nearly every case.

They also stated that "this method may well be the basis of the future treatment of infantile paralysis."[16] Within two years, Sister Kenny's methods had become the dominant form of treatment for polio. She became famous and people swarmed about her wherever she went. But, while her results were clearly better than what had been reported previously, there remained many skeptics in the medical community. Many were openly hostile, and it often was difficult

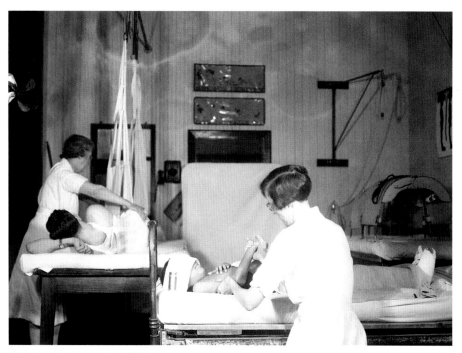

Physical therapy, circa 1940

to determine if they didn't like her treatment ideas or just didn't like her. Another committee of doctors was formed to evaluate her methods, with Dr. Ralph Ghormley as chairman. Melvin Henderson's successor as head of the department of orthopaedic surgery at the Mayo Clinic, Ghormley once had worked with Dr. Robert Lovett. This committee also did not support Kenny. Their conclusions also were published in *The Journal of the American Medical Association.* A committee member, speaking at the American Medical Association meeting in 1944, summed them up: "This report proves that what is good in the Kenny treatment is not new, and what is new is not good."[17]

Kenny was intensely frustrated by the response from the medical community. She had been extremely suspicious of the Ghormley committee when they

visited Minneapolis General Hospital and Gillette State Hospital. She had not been on her best behavior, which did not help her cause. She complained to Dr. Cole about the treatment she received in medical journals.

> The tragedy of inaccurate and untruthful statements published in the medical journals is too well known to you to need repetition. However, the fact that these statements were signed by Dr. Ralph Ghormley, who gave his status as attached to the University of Minnesota Medical School, had a very damaging effect throughout the whole world, for it was known that I was attached to the University, and this was supposed to be an official presentation of two years'

observation. I trust I shall be pardoned if I state that it was the work of a very clever trickster.[20]

She repeated her motivation for coming to the United States.

My only desire is to give to the people of the United States of America every atom of knowledge concerning the disease [of] infantile paralysis which may be in any way effective in bringing about its conquest. . . . I am quite willing to have the epithets of being obdurate, obstinate and all the rest of it hurled at me until I have transmitted my entire knowledge to a reliable group.[18]

Sister Kenny owed a large part of the acceptance she received to Wallace Cole and John Pohl. They were willing to listen, and they accepted her new ideas when they were useful. In particular, Dr. Cole, as a leader among orthopaedic surgeons in the United States, risked his own reputation. This did not seem to bother him. Writing years later, he said:

Unfortunately, there are members of our profession who do not remember how some of the great advances in medical science came about. . . . It is pertinent to quote Oliver Wendell Holmes, who stated that medicine learned "from a Jesuit how to cure agues, from a friar how to cut for stone, from a soldier how to treat gout, from a sailor how to keep off scurvy, from a postmaster how to sound the Eustachian tube, from a dairy maid how to prevent smallpox, and from an old market woman how to catch the itch-insect." In all

Science having proved my revolutionary theory concerning the symptoms of the disease to be correct, I am now in a position to cooperate with anyone desiring such cooperation, and will give them all the help I can.

Elizabeth Kenny
1950

Sister Kenny changed the whole thing. She came out to the hospital, a big lady with broad shoulders who walked like a top sergeant. Dr. Cole said that she could look at his patients, and she went into the ward. I left the office, as I was only twenty feet away. She went up to the first bed, who was a little girl. She would work with her thumb, and the doctors that were with her were just flabbergasted. She told them to put the splints in the trash. By Wednesday of the next week those girls were far ahead of the kids that were in the splints. All of the splints came off.

Dr. Grace Jones
1994

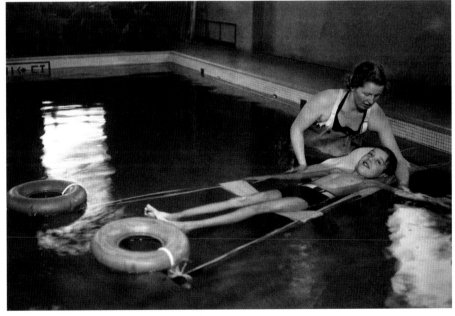

Physical therapy in the pool, circa 1940

97

humility, I suggest that the following be added: "and from an Australian nurse how to treat infantile paralysis."[19]

For fifty years, polio dominated Gillette State Hospital for Crippled Children. No condition before or since brought as many children in for care. For the hospital, polio was like a huge tidal wave that overwhelmed everything in its path. It began in 1917 when children from the 1916 epidemic began to be admitted. Before 1916, no more than thirty-three children with polio were admitted in a single year. In 1917,

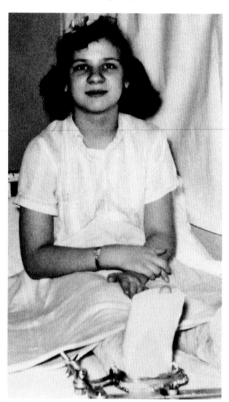

Lois Abramson with her fingers crossed, 1951

106 children were admitted. Thereafter, admissions steadily increased. There was a brief lull in the early years of World War II due to travel restrictions which prevented many young patients from reaching the hospital. In 1946, when travel eased, the hospital was confronted with a backlog of cases. In that year alone, 321 youngsters with polio were admitted. Paralleling national experience, admissions to Gillette State Hospital for the treatment of polio reached their peak in the early 1950s.[20]

In 1952 Dr. Jonas Salk of Pittsburgh began field trials of new vaccines developed in his laboratory and made from individual strains of polio viruses that had been killed by formalin. The vaccines were administered by needle injections, and a new "shot" was required for each new vaccine. Salk's vaccines proved effective, and the number of new polio cases plummeted. In 1961 an oral vaccine made of live "attenuated" polio viruses was developed by Dr. Albert Sabin. Though living, the ability of the viruses to cause illness had been removed. The Sabin vaccine quickly replaced the Salk vaccine and was administered in doctor's offices and school cafeterias across the United States.[21]

At Gillette State Hospital the result was a steady decrease in the number of children with polio. After 1972 no more than

twenty new cases were seen in any one year and most of them were children who had been adopted from Asia, Africa, and India, where polio is still active. Recently some of the survivors of the epidemic years have begun to report signs that the weakness of polio is growing worse in their later adult years. For them, polio is not a thing of the past. It is still here, and just as confusing as it was when it first struck. Lois (Abramson) Johnson, who lives in Meadowlands, Minnesota, describes it well.

I limp but I can get around good, although now with post-polio syndrome we are all starting to get back to these devices that we gladly threw away years ago. . . . I am so much weaker than I used to be. [I always] wake up tired in the morning. It seems like I can't get enough rest. I know the muscles are so much weaker. . . . Of course, the first doctor that I went to told me I was getting older. Funny you should be happy when you hear a diagnosis, finally knowing it's post-polio syndrome. Not that I was happy it was post-polio syndrome, but at least it had a name, and it wasn't in my head.[22]

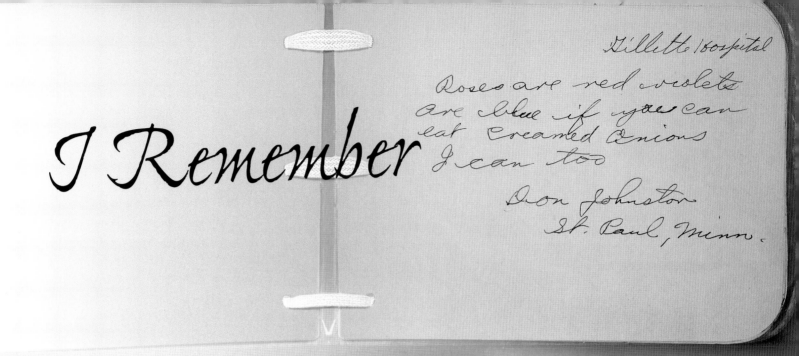

I Remember

Gillette Hospital

Roses are red violets
are blue if you can
eat creamed onions
I can too

Don Johnston
St. Paul, Minn.

Paintings that depict scenes from the rural Midwest during the middle part of this century have become popular. They are often done in warm, soft colors chosen to create a nostalgic longing for a simpler time in American life. The good things are emphasized; the bad things are not shown. It is tempting to portray the lives of the children and staff at Gillette State Hospital for Crippled Children during that time in the same way. All the positive things could be dutifully reported, all the negative things could be gracefully ignored. But that would not be accurate. Life at the hospital was much more complicated than that.

Today we assume that orthopaedic surgeons are able to reshape, repair, or replace those parts of the skeleton that are deformed, injured, or worn out. And we want the work done quickly, with as little intrusion in our busy lives as possible. This was not the experience of children with orthopaedic problems in the earlier years of this century. Many deformities went untreated or were managed with casts, braces, and therapy because surgery was dangerous, unreliable, and painful. Anesthesia was crude, infections were common, blood transfusions were very rare, and metal implants like plates, screws, and rods were being developed. A decision to perform surgery was not made lightly, and recovery from the procedure could take weeks or months.[1]

Thirty to seventy years after their childhood experiences at the hospital, the memories of adults who spent time there vary widely. Consider Lowell Erdahl and Nelvin Vos. Nelvin, later a professor of English at Muhlenberg College in Pennsylvania, was a happy eight-year-old from rural Chandler, Minnesota, in 1940 when he broke his arm and injured the nerves to his hand. Fifty-three years later he remembered his time at the hospital.

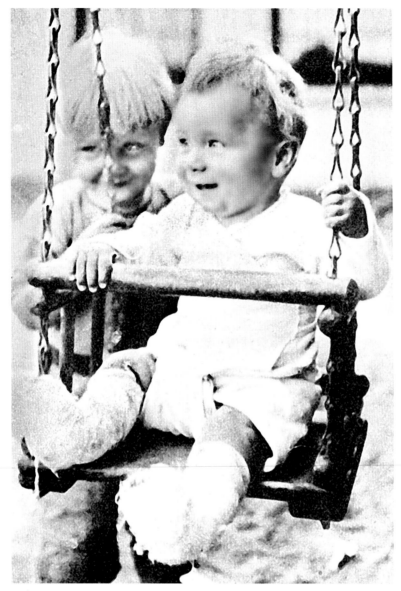

Baby enjoying swing, circa 1920

I learned the necessity of working with others, or, as I would put it now, the sense of community. Most of all, I perhaps began to see what love for others meant and what their love meant to me. Compassion was a word not used in Gillette Hospital. Yet a spirit of compassion took hold there amid the hectic camaraderie.[2]

Lowell, who became a bishop of the Lutheran Church, was two years old and living with his family on a farm near Blue Earth, Minnesota, when he developed polio. He was five years old when he was admitted to Gillette for the first time. Fifty-eight years later his memories were not as positive.

> I did not like being here.
> I hardly ever had any visitors.
> . . . It was much more

traumatic emotionally than it was physically, and it was sufficiently traumatic physically. . . . I am sure that I have emotional scars on my psyche as well as physical scars on my soma from having gone through that experience. One thing that I would say, if I put a positive twist on it, is that I think that it has given me a lot of empathy for people who have various difficulties in life.

The memories of both men are accurate. For some children, their time at Gillette was a bad experience. For others, it was extremely positive. It is important for us to listen to those experiences and to learn from them. The memories of those hospitalized between 1930 and 1960 seem to cluster around certain people or events. The bad experiences were separation from parents, loneliness, surgery and pain, food, the behavior of hospital staff members, and going home to strangers. The good experiences included seeing and learning new things, making friends with other children, being treated well by staff members, eating good food, and going home.

Traveling to the hospital was difficult for Roger Gunderson, who was admitted several times between 1931 and 1952 to treat legs that were paralyzed when his spinal cord was injured at birth. He dreaded the trip from Duluth to St. Paul.

You would have an idea that this was the time you would probably have to stay, so . . . I would really start to get a depressed feeling, almost to the point of crying when I got further in by Phalen Park. I practically knew every step of the way and . . . I would just be a basket case. And, if you were not admitted and you could go back home, you would have such a euphoric feeling.

Lois (Abramson) Johnson grew up on a dairy farm in northern Minnesota, where she contracted polio at age seven. She was admitted to Gillette State Hospital five times between 1950 and 1955. Each trip to the hospital caused her to worry.

"I was always on my guard, because whenever we had a check-up . . . I never knew until I got here if I was going to have to stay or not. My mom used to say that weeks before my appointment I would just sort of change personality at home. I would just sort of clam up and didn't eat normal because I was always worried that I would have to stay."

Occasionally, when younger children were admitted, their parents were advised to leave quickly, without saying goodbye. That was bad advice. Lowell Erdahl remembered the results.

After having been left at the hospital I recall asking a staff member when my parents were coming back and being told that they would return

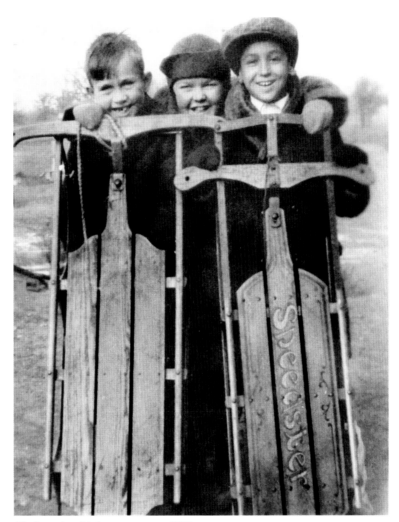

Sleds and cold, but no snow, 1929

about five o'clock. After repeatedly asking about the time, five o'clock came and went and I realized that they had gone home. I now see this event as perhaps my first experience of "loss of innocence."

Parents were hurt by the departure, too. Nancy Radtke was twelve years old when she was admitted for treatment of polio, and her parents were grateful: "We certainly appreciated that she could receive the care needed, as we were a struggling young couple at the

time." But Nancy's mother, Reba, hated leaving her at the hospital.

My memories are not pleasant. In fact, I get tears in my eyes and am choked up on the infrequent occasions I am reminded of it. . . . I will never forget the devastation I felt to walk out of that building and leave her there alone. It had a very adverse effect on her, too.

Once the children were there, they had to adapt to life without their families. That was not easy for Martha (Young) Ignaszewski, who came from a farm in Wells, Minnesota, and was admitted for polio care at age twelve: "I was scared. Scared stiff, I suppose. Homesick. I cried, and I cried, and I cried." For other children, the loneliness was less severe. Mary (Luce) Novak, who came to the hospital from Shakopee, adapted fairly quickly. She was five years old when she was admitted for the first time to treat her polio, and was admitted seven times between 1946 and 1958: "Maybe the first couple of days you were lonesome, but you got to know the other kids, and [then] it was okay. I knew that they were going to be there for a while, too."

The rare visits by parents or family were one of the biggest causes of loneliness. Every adult remembered that they wished they could have seen their family more often. Although visiting hours were scattered throughout the week, the hours were not gener-

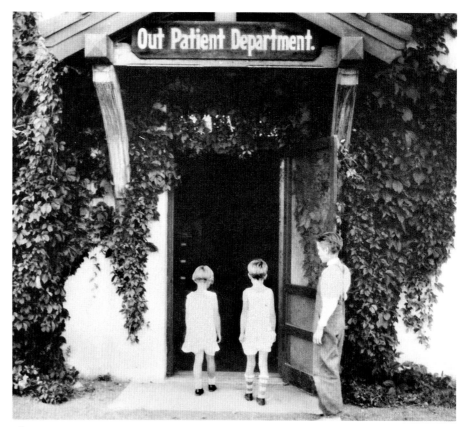

The Outpatient Department, circa 1940

ous, and brothers and sisters were not allowed to visit patients. In addition, many parents lived far away at a time when automobile travel was not easy. One child from southern Minnesota was admitted eleven times between 1953 and 1964 for treatment of his dislocated hips. He was two years old when he was admitted the first time, and his mother remembered being separated from him: "We could look at him through the glass, but never touch him for all that time. . . . None of his siblings were even allowed to see him or come to the hospital. We always waited until we were outdoors before we broke down and cried."

Alfred Gardner developed polio at age seven and later injured his weakened leg in an accident on the family farm near Freeborn, Minnesota. He remembered a visit from his parents when he was in isolation with

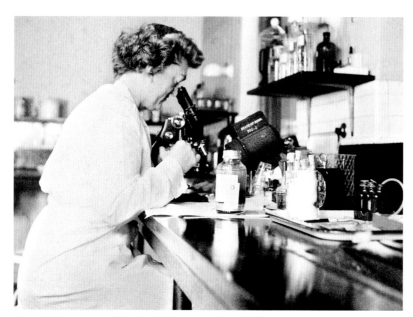

A technician at work in the laboratory, circa 1950

mumps in 1934: "They came and visited me a couple of times. One time I was in isolation and then they had to talk to me from the lawn up to the upstairs window."

The hospital staff was not very flexible about visiting hours. Karen (Oberg) Valerius's parents discovered this one Christmas, when the children were allowed two visitors on one of two days: "My parents misinterpreted the letter and thought I could have two visitors twice. They came on the first day. When my aunt and uncle who had come to see me from Dallas, Texas, came the next day, they were turned away." Karen was admitted ten times between 1946 and 1951, and she learned to beat the system: "When I was a teenager, my girlfriends would dress up with high heels, make-up, and gloves so they could pass for eighteen. Another way to get around the restrictions when I was older was to go outside where more than two friends would cross over the lawn rather than coming in the door."

The children hated blood tests and visits to the dentist. Richard Foley, who lived on a farm near Finlayson, was admitted at age fifteen after his broken arm healed in the wrong position.

I was scared spitless of needles. I still hate the damn things. I refused any hypos or anything after surgery. In fact, I threw water glasses and emesis basins and everything when they tried to give me hypos.

Karen (Oberg) Valerius also dreaded needles.

Thursday was also the day the "stick lady" came. She gave all the blood tests and vaccinations that had been ordered that week. It was a horrible day. She usually came after lunch, but one could never tell when you would hear the tell-tale rattle of her cart coming down the hall. Those needles and syringes [clanging] against the stainless steel containers was a particular sound I will never forget. . . . She began to call off the victims of the day. There was no escape if your name was called. You would be found, under the covers, behind the curtains, in the bath-room. . . . I spent several Thursday afternoons hidden behind the clothes rack in the closet.

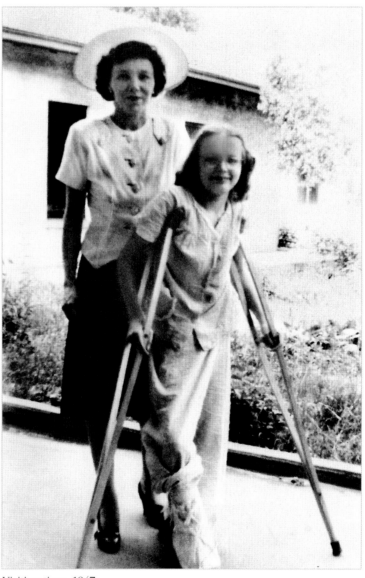

Visiting time, 1947

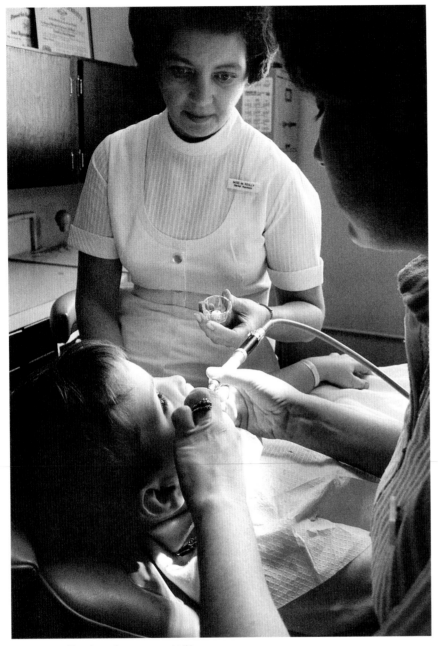

Monica Reilly, dental assistant, 1965

Children were rarely fond of dentists then, and the children in the hospital were no exception. Kathleen (Papenheim) Ramirez, who grew up in St. Paul, liked dental assistant Monica Reilly, but feared Dr. Grace Jones.

> I remember Monica. She was there for most of my life.

Monica was great. I remember the old dentist, too. I don't remember what her name was, but, oh yes, I can even picture her in my mind. She scared me. I was always afraid that she was going to do something to me. . . . I always told my mom to tell her that I just went to the dentist. She scared me. I had heard horror stories about her. I don't know if they were always true, but kids would say things.

Surgery was a frightening experience that left deep memories. Betty (Bowman) Atwood, who grew up in Crow Wing County, went to surgery seven times in thirteen years for problems related to spina bifida. She remembered the ether and the pain after surgery.

> I was held down while an ether mask was put over my face as I struggled. There was an awful smell of rubber and ether and a sensation of spinning faster and faster into a deeper and deeper dark hole. After the surgery they gave me hypos if I said I hurt. When they gave me hypos I would vomit, have bad dreams and nightmares, and couldn't wake up. So I stopped telling them that I hurt.

Richard Olson also remembered the ether.

> The only thing I can remember is the terrible smell of ether. . . . The wrenching sickness that appeared after I woke up from surgery [was] because of the ether. I don't remember too much pain. Either I was well-medicated, or it didn't bother me too much. Too busy being sick!

There was an involved preparation process for surgery. Besides blood tests, it included a bath, shaving of the surgical area, and a warm soap-water enema, which was particularly annoying.[3] On one occasion a surgery planned for Karen (Oberg) Valerius was canceled without explanation: "I threw an absolute fit and told him I was ready for surgery, and they had better do it. They did. My reasoning was, I had already had that enema and I was not going to go through that for nothing."

At that time, tonsils were considered a bad thing, so one of the most common surgeries at Gillette was tonsil and adenoid removal. Tonsils were removed if they looked too large or if a child had a history of throat infections.[4] Some of the children knew about it and tried to avoid the surgery. George Hofford of Two Harbors tried a particularly creative story when he was five years old.

> The doctor told me to open wide, and he peered within. "Have you ever had your tonsils out?" inquired the physician. "Uh huh," I replied. "Who took them out?" queried the physician. "My dad." "And where did he take them out?" the physician prompted. Now here was a dilemma. Should I tell the doctor it was done in the kitchen, or outside? I responded, "It was on the back porch, with the pliers." My guile did not save me, and shortly thereafter I found myself in surgery.

Some children would do anything to avoid surgery. In 1932, while hospitalized for a bone infection, ten-year-old Carolyn Ann (Ekelin) Freeberg of North Branch wrote a letter home to her sister. She described the excitement of the day.

> Dear Grace, . . . This morning while the night nurses were still on, the girls in the porch began to holler, "Miss Holm, Miss Holm, come here quick." The nurse ran out there and they all began to talk at once. "A boy from Ward 5 jumped [out] and ran!" The nurse just smiled and said she didn't believe it. But the children were so sure of it and nobody said "no" and they crossed their hearts, so she went and told the Ward 5 nurse. Then we saw a nurse run after him. There were so many plants and trees we could not see. Pretty soon another nurse ran off to tell somebody because she didn't come back. In a few minutes the nurse and the boy came back walking slowly. The boy had casts on both feet but he walked without limping. He only had his nightgown on. When they came nearer another nurse came out with a wheelchair and the boy sat down and they pulled him in and I haven't seen him since. They said he must not be right in his head, or he was walking in his sleep. After awhile the

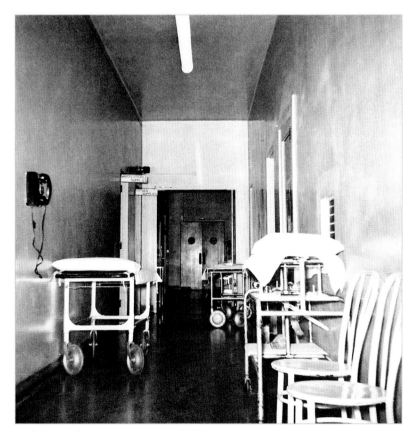

Hallway to the operating room, 1957

nurse that took him in came in our ward and they asked if he was crazy. She said, "No, he tried to run away because he is going to have an operation today. He's in his senses, I'm sure." This afternoon the girls found out he had been operated on anyway. I hear some strong hollering in Ward 5 now. I bet it's him.

The behavior of the nurses and therapists left vivid memories.

Most were positive, but the negative memories lingered for years. Larry Hayes was nine when he came to the hospital from northern Minnesota for treatment of his polio. He remembered a nurse in his ward.

I had a bad experience with a head nurse. If she treated young ones like I was treated by her, and some of the other kids, she would be in a lot of trouble today. . . . I remember

her giving haircuts with the old hand clippers and she would go up your head faster than she was clipping and pulling the hair out. If you yelled she would slap you. There were other things she also did like hitting the kids or sitting [you] on the toilet until you went even if you did not have to go.

Richard Holt of Duluth had polio at age five. He remembered the advice a nurse gave him when he was trying to learn how to walk again.

I would stumble and fall. It seems to me that there was something along the hallway that I would hang on to. The nurse would tell me rather bluntly that I had to get up because there was nobody in life to help me so that I had to get up and walk. I have very vivid memories of that. . . . I don't think that one understands the whole statement that there would be nobody there in life to help you, but the fact that she would not help me right at the time seemed to hurt.

One woman, many years later, came to believe she had been abused by a nurse. She sought help from a mental health professional to work through her memories. Another woman wrote to the hospital forty-three years after her discharge, seeking information about her stay. She was suffering from depression, and one

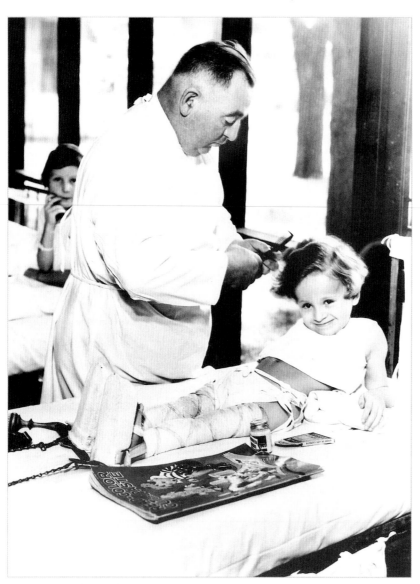

Haircut by volunteer barber, circa 1945

of her doctors had suggested that her long stay in the hospital as a child had created problems. Her plea is heart-wrenching.

> I've had a complete breakdown of the central nervous system and I feel so worthless, unloved, and I am so scared of life and of people, and it is like I don't know all the reasons why I'm scared, or what I'm scared of, and the doctors think some of the answers to the causes of my illness started in the hospital from the trauma of being left alone at four years of age.

Richard Halverson became a ward of the state after he was born with numerous deformities of his legs. He spent the first four years of his life at the hospital, and divided the rest of his childhood between foster care and additional stays in the hospital. He came to see the schedules and routines as necessary and thought it might have strengthened him.

> I think, at least for some of us, we became independent, and I notice that . . . the ones that had the closest family ties . . . and had more people to cater to them did not do as well as the ones that I see like myself, who fought every inch of the way. . . . I don't think the strictness then was any different than the culture of the time.

Many children remembered being punished by being isolated

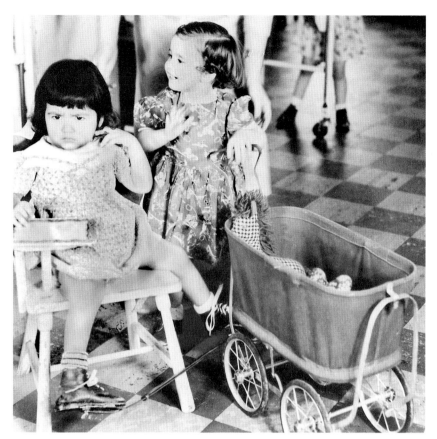

One buggy, two little girls, circa 1960

or by having something taken away. Sometimes the radio or television in the ward was turned off for the night, or toys were put away early. Some of the doctors were impersonal or insensitive. Clair DeVries, from Hollandale, Minnesota, was a polio patient at the age of ten.

> I guess one thing that I remember was that, at that time, you were almost like you were part of the process. It's like you really weren't a person so much, you were a thing to operate on or a thing to study. Well, like you would go in for checkups and you would have ten people walk in and they talk

to everybody but you. Talk back and forth about you, and it seemed like nobody ever really was interested in letting you know what's going on.

Eight-year-old Karen (Bruber) Boche, from South St. Paul, had similar experiences when she was treated for polio.

> I would sit on this table and then they would come in with six or seven doctors around me. They would all examine me. They were not real personable. They talked over my head. They talked about me, but not to me. They had me walk, and they would talk about the way I walked. I did

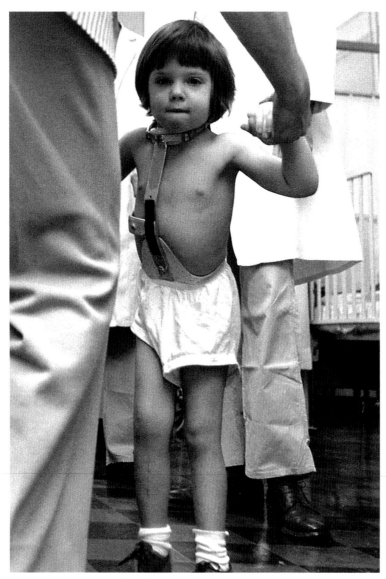

Young patient in a Milwaukee spine brace, 1970

sorts of interesting things to the hospital. The girls sent for free samples of make-up and spent time making each other up. They learned to take care of each other. Healthier children were assigned to help those who were sick or bedridden. When they were lonely, they turned to their neighbor. Richard Foley remembered the boy in the next bed.

> At nine o'clock the lights went out, but we would lay and talk a lot with our next door bed partner. The one boy that was close to me, he was in a body cast from polio and we used to lay and talk a lot, talk about things in school, things we'd like to become and just sympathize with each other. When he . . . had a lot of pain we'd pull our beds together and I'd just lay there and hold his hand and talk to him when he cried and stuff because of the pain.

George Hofford was frightened by lightning.

> Once, when they were showing the film "Pinocchio," there was a scene depicting a lightning storm. [When I began] to cry, the attendant placed me in the lap of one of the biggest boys seated in a wheelchair. I had been afraid of this biggest boy, and he held me and we became friends.

Lifelong friendships began in the hospital. Linda (Fasching) Ruhland of Montgomery developed

not even know what they were saying. I was extremely embarrassed, and that is a lot of why I did not want to come back. I will never forget that.

To Richard Halverson it seemed that the patients in the clinic were not a top priority.

> If your doctor was doing some surgeries he probably didn't start seeing patients until afternoon, and, of course, you sat there. . . . It was a matter of a parent or guardian trying to sit with an ornery little kid all day long and wait, wait, wait.

However, many children had positive experiences. They often turned to each other for support, and they found ways to break up the monotony. When the mail didn't bring letters from home, they answered ads they found in magazines. That would bring all rickets because her body could not form vitamin D properly. She remembered the help she received from another girl there when she was a teenager.

I went through a "feel sorry for myself" period and I thought I was the only one born with a disability. I didn't stop to look around me long enough to see what other people were even in the hospital for. One of the greatest inspirations at that time was Dottie Werner. She had so many problems to deal with and she always had a smile for everyone and something good to say to people around her. Everyone liked her. I just didn't understand her attitude but I studied her hard, and I wanted to learn to be just as positive. She once told me to knock the chip off my shoulder and to make the most with what I had. At least, she said, I could walk which was more than many [including her] could ever do. I looked up to Dottie a lot and she became my close friend.

The buildings and grounds also created some happy memories. Betty (Bowman) Atwood enjoyed the porch.

Some of the best things about Gillette were the screened-in porches between the wards in the summertime. The sun porches at the ends of the wards were nice, too, because you could see outside. The building, location, and grounds at Gillette were wonderful. The lawns were beautiful, with big shade trees. We could watch the man mow the lawns. Sometimes you could smell the cut grass. Lots of squirrels ran between the trees. In the winter, I could see the snowflakes float down, or blow like a blizzard. The men would clean out the circle drive in front of the office, and clear the sidewalks. . . . I think hospitals should have large windows with magnificent views, [where] people can see sun, rain, snow, birds, flowers, and life. I'm sure we'd all get well faster and have a better frame of mind.

Mary Ann (Carlin) Mulcrone was one of eleven children, and grew up on a farm near Foley, Minnesota. She was badly burned when a pot of boiling water tipped over on her. Occasionally she would escape outdoors at night to feel the grass and breathe in the fresh air. She paid a price for doing so.

I would put my washcloth in the door so it wouldn't lock behind me, and I would go out onto the lawn. It was my great joy. I ran and jumped and rolled in the cool grass. The sky was like the sky on the farm. When the grass was freshly mowed it smelled like the farm. It was nothing short

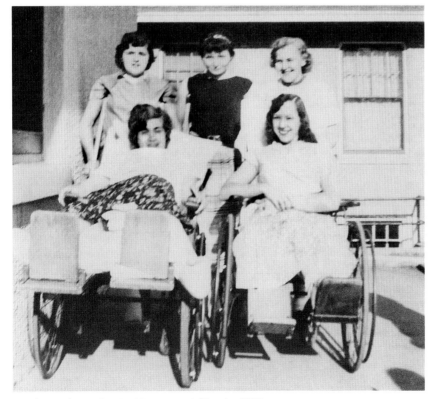

Linda Fasching, Dottie Werner, and friends, 1959

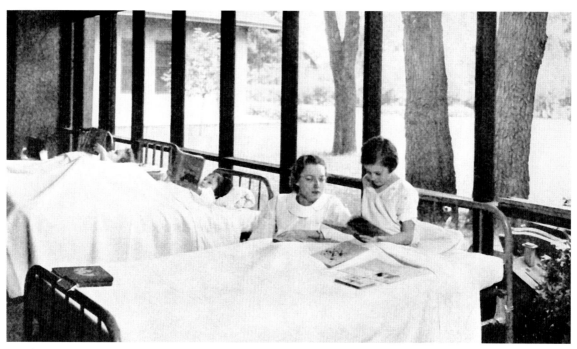

Reading in screened porch, circa 1935

of exhilarating. And I was so happy knowing I was keeping my legs from shrinking or twisting up, and my feet from falling off. . . . One day, after rainy weather, I had slightly muddy feet. I dampened my washcloth with my glass of water and carefully wiped my feet off. I forgot about the filthy cloth being a dead give-away. I was caught! They threatened me but I kept sneaking out. They didn't catch me again for awhile, but when they did they moved me to another cubicle and tied me to the bed. That was a devastating setback for me.

At other times, members of the staff were wonderfully sensitive. Karen (Oberg) Valerius, whose polio had weakened one of her legs, remembered a special kindness from Dr. Cole.

Dr. Cole ordered an artificial calf for my leg when I asked him to do something about the difference in the size of my legs. They developed a molded piece of foam rubber that had to be glued on and covered with a tight elastic stocking. It did not work well, but they had the compassion to try to soothe my teenage vanity.

Some people remembered being very involved in the decisions that were made about medical treatment. Elizabeth Reimann remembered what her late husband, Michael, who grew up in Minneapolis, said about the medical discussions about his leg. He was born with severe shortening of his left leg, and it was difficult for his doctors to determine what treatment would be the best.

The thing that he mentioned that kind of stuck in my mind was the decision process of what to do. "His leg [is] so short, do we cut the foot off since it is [at] knee level, or turn that foot around and make the heel look like a knee? Cosmetically it would be more acceptable, but this is a joint decision." Another doctor would say "No, he's got the feel of his foot, the depth perception in his toes and I think that is important," and then looking to his parents and saying, "What do you think?" Genuinely listening to them . . . not just one doctor making the decision and then the family comes in a month later and sees what happened.

Usually the children were thrilled to go home to their families.

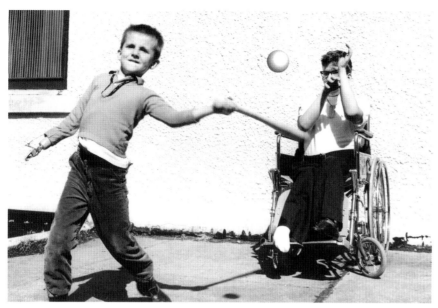

Boys playing baseball, circa 1960

Minnesota, was able to use a special talent.

The Bible says that all things work together for good to those who love Him and are called according to his purpose. What has that good been? The doctor recommended that I learn to play the piano to help with my coordination. So, around the age of eight, I began lessons which continued through high school. The Lord blessed my piano playing over the years. A high school highlight for me happened when I returned to school following my surgery as a junior. The choir had been practicing a number for a contest that was to be held in a few days. The piano part was very difficult, so one boy played the treble clef and one boy played the

Some children were less sure. One person put the dilemma this way: "Was I going home, or was I leaving home?" For Arliss (Klevenberg) Godejohn there was no doubt that home was with her family in rural Cyrus, Minnesota: "The hardest thing is being away from your parents and brothers and sisters. I loved to ride horseback and loved to be outdoors." Her doctor told her she could ride a horse when she got home, if she was able to get up on it. She wasted no time: "I went and caught my horse and I took him in the barn, and I'll bet you it took me an hour or an hour and a half to get on that horse, but I did it."

Fifteen-year-old John Tobish got together with his old friends when he went home to the east side of St. Paul. He had been admitted when a growth area in the ball of his hip slipped out of place: "When we would go out to swipe apples and plums I could get the bigger and better ones by using my crutches to reach the ones higher up in the trees. Swiping apples was a favorite pastime with the kids in our neighborhood."

Beverly (Dixon) Krueger, who developed polio as an infant on the family farm near Princeton,

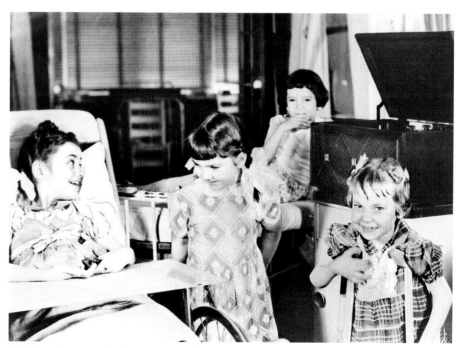

Enjoying the record player, circa 1960

bass clef. It was not going well. I knew I could do it, but was afraid to say anything. Then my friends cornered me and asked if I could play it. What a thrill to show those two boys I could do it by myself.

As they grew older, some of the children had very appropriate fears about how they would fit into society, and whether anyone would love them. Mary (Bloom) Newman of St. Paul had to work through some difficult experiences with her spina bifida.

Dating and slumber parties or staying overnight was never a reality. It was so painful to hear all the nasty jokes [or be] bombarded with questions, not being able ever to reveal my secret of wearing diapers, dreadful embarrassing moments of accidents I had because of little or no bladder and bowel control. And even after my diversion, having to wear a pouch, I never dreamed there'd be a man who would love me beyond the physical presence I would expose if we should ever become intimate.

Mary did find a man who would love her. They were married in 1972 and have two daughters, but it was not easy for her to believe she was lovable.

It was a problem for me to accept that he loved me unconditionally. When I was growing up I never, truthfully, I never felt I would find someone that I could marry because, of course, of my problem and because I have so many embarrassing moments. What man in the world would ever even look at someone like me, much less think about marrying.

But not every dream came true. Many patients had to adapt to limitations during their adult years. Betty (Bowman) Atwood had one or two things she wished she could have done: "I regret my inability to ride a bicycle and shovel dirt for my gardening. If I wasn't handicapped, I think I would have enjoyed walking the Appalachian Trail. I think we all have dreams."

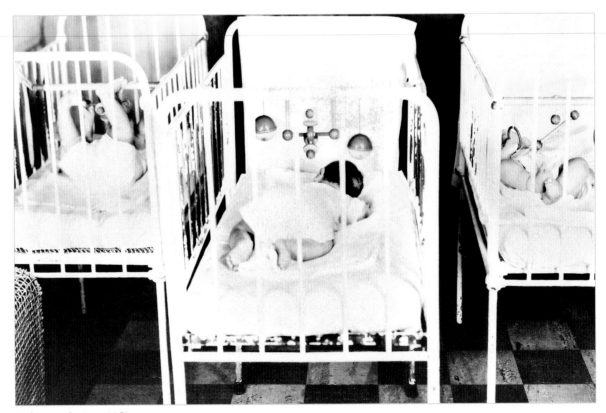

Baby ward, circa 1960

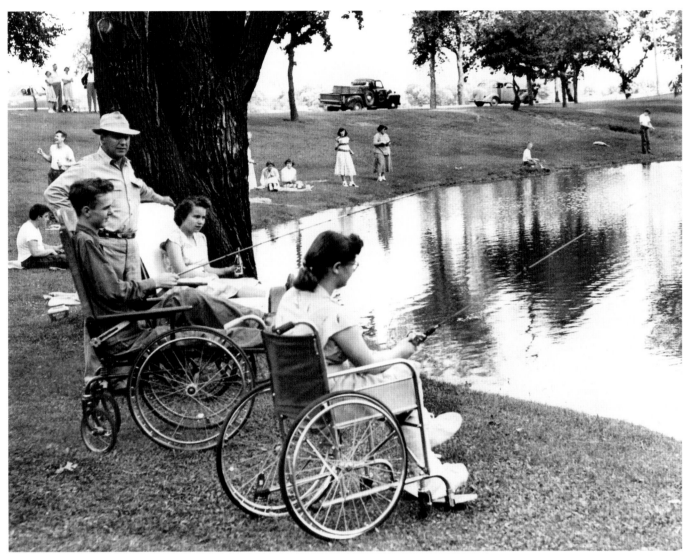

Fishing at Phalen Creek, circa 1950

Some children learned perspective during their stay in the hospital. Marlene Gardner's understanding of her cerebral palsy was changed by her experience.

I think maybe I probably felt sorry for myself when I was little because I couldn't do these things. But, you know, I've never taken anything for granted since the first day I walked into Gillette. . . . I was an abnormal person in a normal world outside, because none of my family or friends had something like what I had. But when I got to Gillette I found out that I was by far better off than anybody else. . . . If I can put it in a nutshell, it gave me a normal life.

Their brothers and sisters were changed, too. Florence Bergvall is the sister of Hazel Howe, who, in 1927 at age eight died of shock after a surgery to remove a bone infection. Florence and Hazel were part of a family of nine children from Cohasset. Almost seventy years later, Florence still thinks of Hazel.

I am sure this was a difficult time for both her and my parents, because times and conditions being what they were, they weren't able to go see her. In fact, when word came she had died, my dad was working in the harvest fields in the Dakotas and the funeral had to be [held] with him gone. I remember the casket laying in the living room at our house and Mom taking my two older sisters and myself in to say good-bye to her. I balked at the request, but that sight is with me today. Mom didn't force me to go in. . . . Among Hazel's meager possessions that were brought home from the hospital was a well-worn doll, not much by today's standards, but a treasure to her. I counted myself lucky to have become the owner of that doll, and only recently gave it to a daughter who is a doll collector. It has a place of honor among her other dolls. My heart goes out to that sick little girl away from home so long ago. It has been like trying to look back into a dim and murky past to talk to my sisters and pull up the memories that are there. I wish I knew more about her.

For some, looking back was an opportunity to look forward. Nelvin Vos carefully measured his past and his future.

My family, my friends, and my students very seldom mention my arm. Is it because they don't notice, or because it's not important, or because they don't know what to ask or say? I find I do now talk about it and my history, when it's appropriate.

A fine wife, three wonderful children, an eighteenth-century stone farmhouse with a very large garden and greenhouse, a half dozen books and many other writings, a Ph.D. from the University of Chicago, the leadership roles at Muhlenberg College, deep involvement in the local, regional, and national church as well as my ecumenical contacts in this country and abroad—such milestones I begin to recognize in this year-long sabbatical leave, especially during the writing of this report.

Sabbatical leaves force one to look back. That is why this exercise was important to me even if none of it is useful to the hospital. Rereading all the correspondence, talking to my mother (my father died in 1983), and most of all, sorting out the experience has been meaningful. Sabbatical times also insistently ask: What next?

I will continue to see service to God and others as critical. And, if I can be instrumental in getting one student to perceive that what one thinks is a liability may really also be an asset, then my disability and my Gillette experience will have served its purpose.

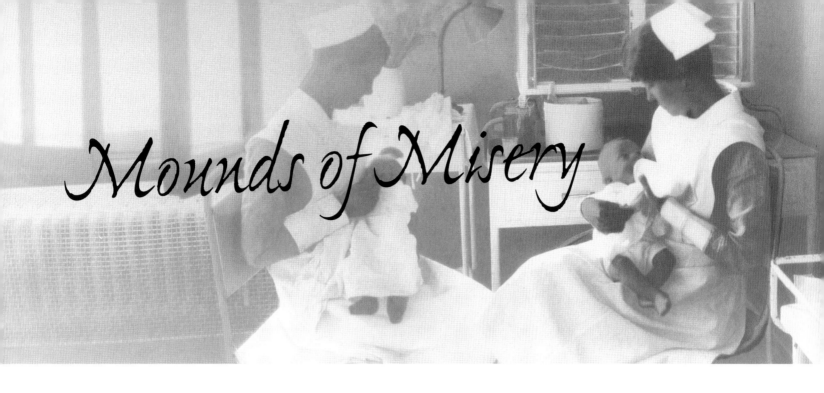

Mounds of Misery

At noon on October 19, 1949, Elizabeth McGregor retired as superintendent. She was seventy-four years old and had served for thirty-five years. At the time of her retirement many of the younger employees and physicians were unaware of the hospital's early history and the vital role she had played in its growth. She was, for many, simply a stern taskmaster. They would have been surprised to learn of the mothers of patients that she had hired, or the past patients she had sent off to school as young adults.

They certainly would not have expected the kindness that she displayed toward a mother who wrote to her in 1920 after reading an article about the hospital in her local newspaper. The woman was touched by a photograph showing five toddlers sunbathing on the lawn of the hospital. One of the children strongly resembled the mother's own child, who had died. She asked Miss McGregor if the child's parents were alive, perhaps hoping they weren't and that the child might need a mother. They were very much alive, and Miss McGregor responded gently:

> In reply to your inquiry about the baby I will say that this child was born with club feet. Her parents are living and want her, of course, as soon as she is ready to leave the hospital. She has been at the hospital since September 1919, and is improving constantly. She is one of the nicest babies and her mother is making the sacrifice of getting along without her, possibly for two years, in order that she may have her deformity corrected. I thank you for your interest, and I think if your baby looked like her, she must have been a very attractive child.[1]

Elizabeth McGregor was succeeded by Jean Conklin. Miss Conklin, as she was known throughout her tenure, was born in Minneapolis on January 28, 1913. She grew up in Bloomington and attended the University of

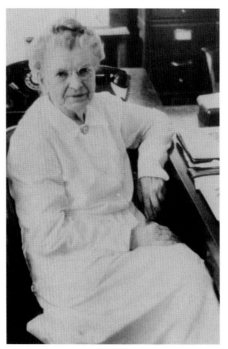

Elizabeth McGregor, 1949

Minnesota for her undergraduate studies. In 1940 she graduated from the Kahler Hospital School of Nursing in Rochester, and then worked as a registered nurse in Cedar Falls, Iowa. A friend who knew of her interest in pediatric nursing told her about an opening at the Gillette State Hospital for Crippled Children and she began work there as the supervisor of pediatric nursing on July 1, 1940. In February 1942 she was granted a leave of absence to enlist in the United States Army Nurse Corps, and during the next four years she served with hospital units in England, Tunisia, and Italy.[2]

When the war ended she returned to Gillette hospital as a nursing supervisor and an instructor in pediatric nursing. She also earned a degree in nursing education from the University of Minnesota in 1947. Most important of all, Elizabeth McGregor took note of

her work. In the summer of 1947 she summoned Jean to her office. Jean remembered the visit clearly.

> She called me into her office and she said, "Won't you sit down, Miss Conklin?" You never sat in her office. You stood at attention. I thought, "My God, this is really going to be terrible. I can't even take it standing up!" So I sat down and I said, "Yes, Miss Elizabeth, what may I do for you?" She said, "I just wanted to tell you that I've selected you as my successor." I said, "What? You don't even know me." "Oh, I've been studying you, and [my sister] Margaret told me about you." I said, "I won't take the job without a degree in hospital administration." "Well," she said, "hurry up and get it. I'm getting tired."

Jean completed the course work for her master's in hospital administration in one year. She was then required to serve a one-year internship, but after Governor Luther Youngdahl and the Commissioner of Public Welfare interviewed her, she was appointed immediately with the proviso that her first two years at Gillette would substitute for her internship. From the start, she brought a different style to the job.

> I took the job on October 19, 1949, with no background. I spent a week with Miss McGregor, and I'll never forget it. She lived in the

same apartment that I lived in for years. The first morning I came out to breakfast I had a blue silk dress on, and she looked at me so funny. I said, "I'm not wearing a uniform. I'm the administrator." She said, "That's your decision. I'll get you a white coat." And I said, "All right." So, she had a little to say about this.

The change in leadership went well. Miss McGregor was gracious and supportive, but Jean knew that changes were needed. She decided to move slowly.

Miss McGregor had been there for thirty-five years. I thought, "You can't come in with a new broom and sweep everything clean." You study it, and you gradually change things and let people become used to you. The first thing I did was to redecorate the hospital. Miss McGregor had gone through the war years with no maintenance money, and nobody to do the maintenance if she wanted it. So, the whole place needed repainting. It was all painted beige, "institutional beige," I called it. So, we put colors in, and new curtains. This kind of alerted the staff that there were going to be some changes. I told Miss McGregor, "I'll be making changes." And she said, "Of course you will." I used to go and pick her up for dinner, and then we'd sit down after dinner and she'd say, "Now,

what have you changed this two week period?" We'd talk it over, and she'd say, "Good, that's great." You know, she was right behind me.

Miss McGregor moved to an apartment in St. Paul but she did not live long after her retirement. She died of a stroke on April 1, 1950, and was buried near her family home at Hawley, Minnesota.[3]

Although they both were extremely effective administrators, Elizabeth and Margaret McGregor did not encourage independent thinking among members of the hospital staff. Even so, Jean Conklin had a deep respect for the McGregor sisters.

Elizabeth was a remarkable person. She was very small, very determined, very autocratic. You never argued with Miss McGregor. You didn't

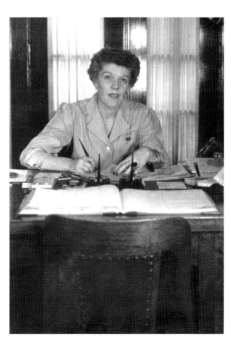

Jean Conklin, 1949

argue with Margaret, either. Elizabeth ran a good hospital. The doctors were gods. Whatever they wanted, they got. She was good with the children, but she didn't spend too much time with them. I think I spent more time with them than she did, but she was good with them. In fact, she was mellow with them. When you saw Elizabeth otherwise, you wondered if it was the same person. Margaret was a little taller, and much fleshier, and very abrupt in her way. She was a good nurse, and very sympathetic, except you didn't realize it until something [bad] happened. Then she'd take care of you, and you knew she was thinking of people. They were quite a pair.

Jean Conklin attempted to instill independent thinking in her staff.

That's one thing that confused the hospital staff when I first came. I delegated duties. With Miss McGregor, you wouldn't pick up a pin without asking her if you could do it first. That's the way they were trained, so that's the way they were going to do it. I said, "No, I'm paying you to assume certain responsibilities. When you find you can't [do something], then you call me and I'll come and help you." It took a while to get them to the point where they'd do it.[4]

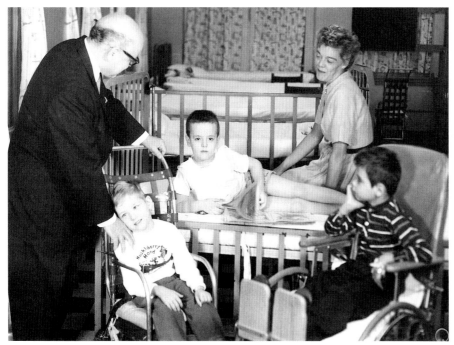
Conklin with patients and a visiting doctor, circa 1950

Janet Hartman, who became the operating room supervisor in 1968, liked Miss Conklin's style.

> Jean Conklin [used] battleship management. She was smart, and she knew the patients and the personnel. You knew where you stood with her, no matter what happened. If you were in the right, she stood behind you, and if you were in the wrong, she told you.[5]

The first changes in hospital routine came in the outpatient department. Since the days of Dr. Gillette most outpatients were seen during clinics held on Thursdays, but this became impractical after World War II. With transportation more readily available, families were able to bring their children for examination and return home the same day. When a stay in the hospital was necessary, some children were sent home in casts and braces with plans worked out to follow their progress during clinic visits. The hospital was slow to respond to this new reality. A letter from a frustrated mother to Elizabeth McGregor in October 1948 described a typical visit and the response of one staff member.

> My husband took time from his work to drive us to the hospital for our nine o'clock appointment, which we made on time. It got to be ten o'clock, so I asked one of your nurses if it would be much longer before we could see the doctors. She replied, "No, they are all here." Patiently, we waited until eleven-thirty. Not realizing that it would take so long, I didn't come prepared with orange juice and her eleven-thirty feeding. With the combination of being hungry, and missing her morning nap, the baby was getting very cross and irritable. Naturally, I approached your nurse again, and asked her if she had any idea of how much longer it would be, as I just had to give this baby some care. She gave me a very abrupt answer, and said it would be sometime after dinner. I told her my appointment was for nine o'clock, and here it was noon, and with the baby it was difficult to wait any longer. Of course, this all led into an argument back and forth.[6]

The physicians were accustomed to the children being admitted to the hospital for their care and they resisted changes in the Thursday clinic, but Miss Conklin pushed hard to make them.

> When I came there the children stayed [in the hospital] for 159 days. That was the average length of stay. When I left, they stayed nine days. I suggested to the doctors that we didn't have to keep the child through his complete convalescence. They said, "What do you mean?" "Well," I said, "Their parents can take care of them. They've got public health facilities out in the state. We've got Crippled Children's Clinics going around. The normal place for a child is in his home."

They said, "They'd never take care of him." And I said, "They will too. Could we try it and see?" "All right, we'll try it, but we don't think it will work." They were so surprised when it did work. Those parents were so happy.

While the medical staff doubted the ability of parents to provide care for their children at home, another factor may have initiated a change in the structure of the clinics. The doctors were beginning to specialize in certain types of problems, and they found it helpful to work together and share their knowledge. It seemed natural to keep children with similar problems together in one clinic. The Thursday clinic was broken up, and clinics were held every weekday.[7] Perhaps the best example of the fruit of

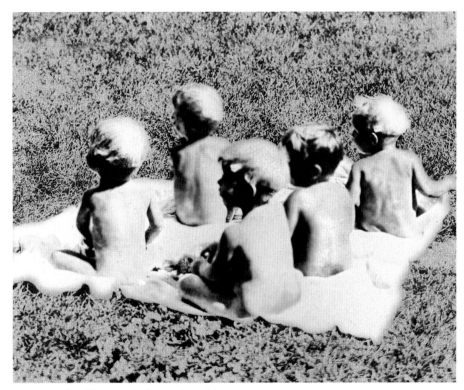

A group of toddlers sunbathing, circa 1920

clinic restructuring was Dr. John Moe's work with children who had developed deformities of the spine.

Every spine has natural curves. The upper back gently rounds outward, and the lower back curves in. Some children develop curves which twist the spine, bending it to the right or left while pushing the ribs out to form large humps. Doctors give these curves names, such as scoliosis, kyphosis, and lordosis. The great majority of these curves remain small and cause few problems. Other children develop severe spine deformities which might change their appearance and cause pain when they become adults. A badly distorted spine and rib cage might even damage the lungs and heart and lead to death as a young adult. For many people,

their curvature is a burden. Irish poet Brendan Kennelly was confronted on the streets of Dublin by a man who had severe scoliosis. Many people with scoliosis would agree with Kennelly's description of that man's experience.[8]

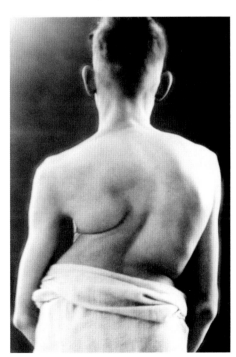

Severe scoliosis with kyphosis, 1923

Day after twisted day,
*   I carry it on*
My back—this devil's hump,
*   this mound*
Of misery sprung from
*   the roots in*
My Body's clay, grotesque
*   companion*
Of my wildest dreams.
*   I have to bend*
Beneath it, flame and rage
Because distortion is
*   my closest friend,*
The faithful ally of my
*   youth and age.*

I walked by this kid's room and he was laying in bed in full body traction with the halo device [attached to his head], and I got really concerned at that point. Am I going to end up like that? I had never seen anything like that . . . that initial twenty minutes of being at the hospital is something I will never forget. . . . .

All of a sudden you have thirty pounds of plaster on you and it's like, "Okay, now what do I do?" Do you feel sorry for yourself or do you try to make the best of it? It's not like . . . six weeks later you get the cast off. We're talking months. It basically can rearrange your life right down to sleeping and bathing. . . . .

I thought it was the greatest thing in the world [when the cast was removed]. I looked down and I could count each rib. There was no meat. It was great!

David Corrin
1994

Some of the kids would start telling you how terrible this would be and it scared me. It was frightening. I just sort of heard rumors that I was going to have a halo cast . . . and it scared me enough that I walked out of the hospital from one of the classrooms and walked home [in St. Paul]. . . .

Donald Oman
1994

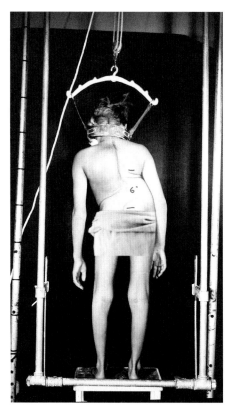

Spine suspension therapy, 1931

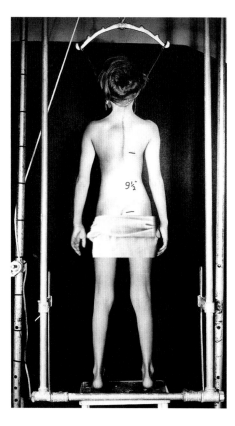

Before 1950 the treatment of childhood spine deformities was largely ineffective. For example, suspension treatment was accomplished by a rope and pulley attached to an overhead frame. The rope was tied to a halter which was placed on the child's head and under the chin while the child stood inside the frame, and the spine was stretched by placing weight on the rope on the other side of the pulley. Jean (O'Reilly) Wright of Goodhue, Minnesota, was fourteen when she was admitted in 1935 for treatment of her scoliosis.

> At first it was exercises. When I was a patient in the hospital they used to hang me by my neck with my toes barely touching the floor. I would hang for what seemed like hours and hours. I don't suppose it was that long. It was not the most fun thing that I ever did.[9]

Corsets, plaster of Paris casts, and braces made of leather were used to support the spine, but many curves worsened. Jean Wright remembered a special cast, called a turnbuckle cast, that was used to straighten bad curves.

> Dr. Cole decided that he would like to try something different on me. He [wanted] to put me in this cast and then split it around the waist and put screws on it and then turn the screws a little bit every day. Luckily, Dr. Williamson came back before Dr. Cole could start this. He vetoed it

and started my surgery much sooner. Instead they put another girl in this thing, and I can still hear her crying.

The first spine fusion surgery in the United States was performed in New York in 1911. Bone was removed from one part of the body and placed along the bones of the deformed spine. The graft caused the bones of the spine to grow together, or "fuse." A fused spine deformity was rigid, but stable. Flexibility was lost in that

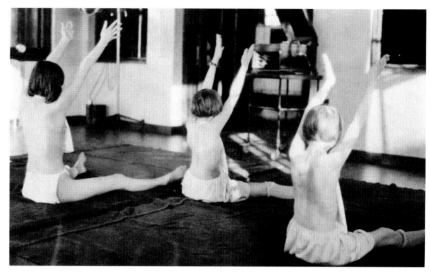
Performing exercises to treat scoliosis, circa 1940

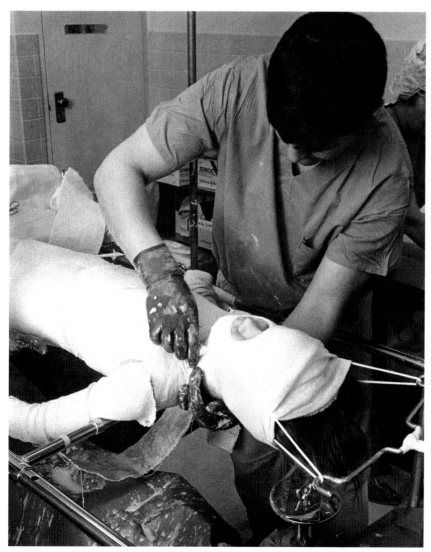
Applying body cast, circa 1970

part of the spine, but the deformity did not worsen. The first fusion surgery in Minnesota was performed at the State Hospital for Indigent Crippled and Deformed Children in 1915, and a second was done in 1916; then it was not attempted again until 1924. Interest in spine fusion surgery reached a peak in 1929, when twenty-three procedures were performed. Then it dropped steadily. From 1942 through 1946 a total of eighteen spine surgeries were performed, but there were none the following year.[10]

Spine surgery before World War II had been filled with dangers, and complications were common. Anesthesia was primitive and unpredictable. The surgery was bloody, and blood transfusion was not reliable. Antibiotics had not been developed, and infections were common. The proper technique for obtaining the bone graft and placing it along the spine had not been worked out, and the desired fusion frequently failed to develop. There were no metal rods or devices to hold the spine straight

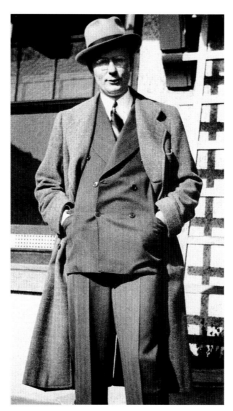

Dr. John Moe, 1939

and still, and children were kept in casts and in bed for months. The results of childhood spine deformity treatment were so dismal that Dr. Chatterton and Dr. Cole were happy to agree to Dr. John Moe's request in 1947 that he be allowed to concentrate on this problem.[11]

John Howard Moe was born on August 14, 1905, on a farm near Grafton, North Dakota, the youngest of the six children of his Norwegian immigrant parents. He attended the University of North Dakota and graduated from medical school at Northwestern University in 1929. After medical school he became interested in orthopaedic surgery, but his education was interrupted when he needed treatment for tuberculosis. In 1932 he arrived at Gillette Children's Hospital as a physician-in-training,

and in 1934, when he decided to stay in the Twin Cities to practice medicine, he was invited to join the hospital's medical staff. For the next fifteen years he took care of children with a wide variety of medical problems. He performed his first spine fusion surgery at the hospital on July 10, 1935, but in the next decade he did only twenty-two more fusion procedures.

Over the span of twenty-five years, beginning with the formation of the Spine Service in 1947, Moe completely changed the surgical treatment of severe deformities of the spine. Several factors helped him succeed where everyone else had failed. His thirteen years as a staff physician leading up to 1947 had given him a broad understanding of the diseases and disorders which caused spine deformities in children. Those years also allowed him to understand Gillette hospital and its staff. He combined a keen ability to analyze problems with a prairie farmer's work ethic to create a system of care which focused on the specific problems of spine deformities.[12]

In the 1950s a typical scoliosis patient was admitted to the hospital several weeks before surgery and a series of plaster body casts were applied in an attempt to straighten the curve as much as possible. Surgery was performed through large openings made in the last corrective cast. This gave the bone graft along the spine a chance to heal without being displaced. After surgery the young patients had to remain in the cast for up to a year, and flat on their backs for the first six months. Many times the bone graft failed to form a solid spine fusion, and the whole process was repeated. Dr. Robert Winter succinctly described the experience for everyone involved: "These casts were a terrible nuisance to put on. They were a terrible nuisance for the patients and the nurses and a huge nuisance in the operating room where it was difficult to have a sterile field during the surgery. We had to have a cast saw plugged in during surgery in case there was a crisis so that we could get the cast off quickly."[13]

After the start of the Spine Service Dr. Moe performed 857 fusion surgeries at Gillette. He was a skillful and creative surgeon, and he was open to change whenever he saw a good idea. He perfected the surgical technique necessary to create a solid fusion, and he was quick to recognize the value of the metal rods that had been developed by Dr. Paul Harrington of Texas in the

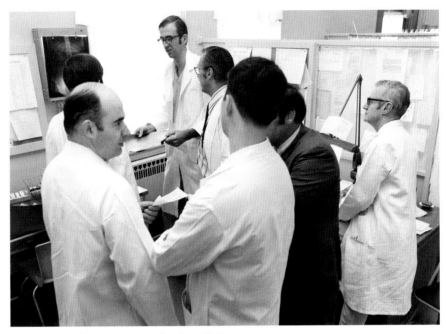
Dr. Winter making spine rounds, circa 1970

late 1950s. Harrington rods were made of stainless steel and were attached to the bones of the spine with metal hooks in order to change the shape of a spine curvature. The first spinal fusion surgeries that included placement of a Harrington rod were performed at the hospital in 1960. Because the rods improved the curves, corrective casts were not necessary before surgery. The rods also provided enough stability for the spine that children were able to stand and walk in their casts shortly after surgery. Moe also helped Drs. Walter Blount and Albert Schmidt of Milwaukee develop a brace which allowed children with some types of scoliosis to be treated without surgery.[14]

Moe's work with children with spine deformities brought him considerable fame. In 1958 he succeeded Dr. Cole as chief of staff at Gillette, and in the same year he became head of the

division of orthopaedic surgery at the University of Minnesota. In 1965 he was one of the founders of the Scoliosis Research Society, and he served as its first president. In 1971 he became president of the American Orthopaedic Association, a position that Dr. Gillette had held in 1900.[15]

Dr. Moe also was a good teacher. Wednesdays became "spine day," when he set aside time to see all the children in the hospital, perform surgery, and instruct the orthopaedic residents. Rather than giving lectures he preferred to have the residents take turns sitting in the "hot seat," a chair in front of an x-ray viewing box. There he helped them analyze cases that demonstrated important principles. One of those residents was Robert Winter.

Robert Winter was born in Cedar Rapids, Iowa, and graduated from Grinnell College in 1954. He attended medical school at

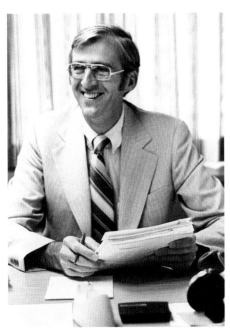
Dr. Robert Winter, circa 1977

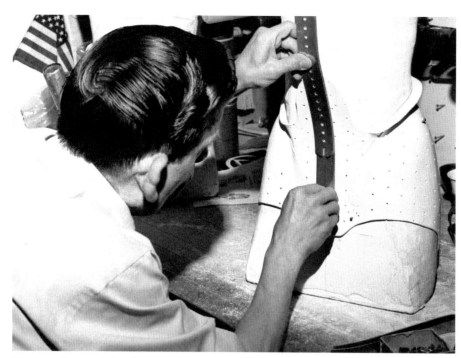

Making a light-weight Milwaukee brace, circa 1970

Washington University in St. Louis, where one of his medical student assignments was the local unit of the Shriners Hospitals. There he saw children with scoliosis being treated with turnbuckle casts, which left him unimpressed with orthopaedic surgeons. In 1958 he began an internship at Minneapolis General Hospital (now Hennepin County Medical Center) and his work on the orthopaedic service changed his opinion. Now interested in becoming an orthopaedic surgeon, he visited Dr. Moe at the University of Minnesota, although he knew nothing of Moe's national reputation. On the day of Winter's interview Dr. Moe gave him a position as an orthopaedic resident. That brought him to Gillette Children's Hospital in 1960 where he impressed Dr. Moe with his hard work and careful attention to the children. Winter finished his residency in 1963 by spending

six months in New Orleans studying hand surgery. He joined a general orthopaedic practice in St. Paul, but Dr. Moe asked him to become a member of the spine service and begin a study of children with congenital spine deformities. This work, and a trip to Brazil in 1966 with Dr. Moe, were turning points in his career.

Dr. Moe's reputation brought him numerous invitations to visit hospitals around the world. In 1966 when he took Winter with him to help establish a scoliosis center in Sao Paolo, Brazil, Moe had been asked to stay for three months, but he knew he could stay only three weeks. He left Winter in charge, with the result that Winter found himself in another "hot seat."

This was a great training experience for me, as we saw nothing but pure pathology in Brazil and were not

encumbered by anything except the problems of the patients. Being left in Brazil to carry on the program, being the one in charge, making all the decisions, and doing all the surgeries was a big responsibility for a young surgeon. It all went pretty well. It gave me a surge of enthusiasm for scoliosis work and the confidence I needed to do this kind of work.

In 1971 Winter dropped his general orthopaedic practice to concentrate full-time on spine deformities, a practice that continued until his retirement in 1995.

Winter had many of Moe's attributes, but he possessed some additional skills. He was an extraordinarily gifted surgeon who knew that hard work was the key to good results for his patients. He possessed a particular talent as a teacher. Early in his career he demonstrated the capacity to take a large body of information, sift it, organize it, and derive knowledge from it that could be applied to future patients. This allowed him to write articles still cited today, and made his teaching conferences invaluable to the resident physicians at the hospital. He also had a capacity for administration. His skills and the need for consistent supervision and teaching of residents were recognized when the job of medical director was created for him. Later he was elected chief of staff by his peers on the medical staff. He became a professor of orthopaedics at the University of Minnesota, and in

1973 he was elected president of the Scoliosis Research Society.[16]

Winter was interested in improving the quality of spine braces for children and this coincided with Jean Conklin's desire to change the brace shop. Together they hired J. Martin Carlson, a young man who would more than satisfy their expectations.

Marty Carlson grew up on a farm near Mora, Minnesota, where he enjoyed the solitude of field work and the endless repair needs of second-hand machinery. In high school he discovered the magic of mathematics, which gave him the ability to solve problems by indirect means. With the start of the space age in the late 1950s he decided on a career in aeronautical engineering. He had been drawn to the mechanical aspects of engineering during college and graduate school, and when he graduated he took a job in research and development with Rosemount Engineering. This gave him a chance to work with technicians and machinists and to understand

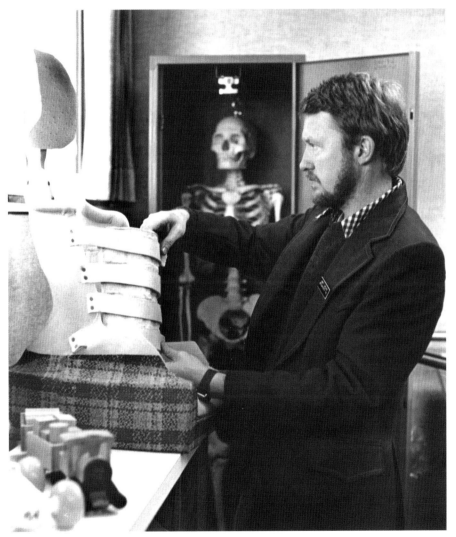

Marty Carlson, brace shop director, circa 1975

I was kind of a thorn in his side. The Milwaukee brace came in, and when they came for outpatient visits they always came up and I looked at their teeth. The first case Dr. Moe had the [child's] teeth were loose. I thought, "Well, that's only one," and I didn't say anything about it. The second time somebody came in their teeth also were loose. Then I started taking plastic impressions of the teeth before they went in [their brace]. When they [returned] I took another impression. Then I would have the two impressions together so that they could look to see how the teeth had moved. He was not very impressed with that.

Dr. Grace Jones
about Dr. Moe, 1994

He was always teaching. He was a man of immense reputation and respect. There was one technique that he had when he taught or lectured that was very unusual. He displayed his mistakes, cases where, in retrospect, he had done the wrong thing or made the wrong decision. That said something, not only about his ability to teach in a way that helped students remember but also about his security as a man and a surgeon.

Marty Carlson
about Dr. Moe, 1996

the development of new products. Still, something was missing and Marty was unhappy with his work.

Except for some other factors, I might have blundered along in "quiet desperation" for many, many years, perhaps throughout an entire engineering career, just feeling that the technical challenge and the livelihood were all I could expect to get out of my work life. Something else was going on during this period which made it impossible for me to continue as I had been. That additional factor was the Vietnam war. I cannot overstate the profound effect that war had on me personally. The images, words, and statistics of the news flooded me [and] I knew that my tax dollars were being spent in support of sustaining that horror. I came to a point where I got more and more desperate to change something in my life so that I could feel I was contributing in a more positive way to human existence. I felt a need to compensate, I suppose, for some of the suffering that, whether I liked it or not, I was connected to through my taxes and my nation. As my desperation grew, I looked for ways to change my career.

His first thought was medical school, but the dean's office at the University of Minnesota suggested

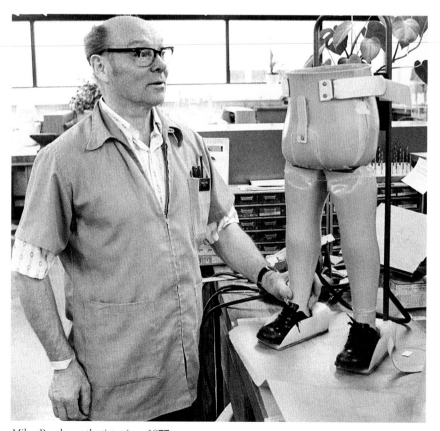

Mike Pearl, prothetist, circa 1977

that at the age of thirty he might be too old. His application for law school was accepted, but he decided that wasn't right for him. One day it occurred to him that artificial limbs required considerable engineering and helped a lot of people. When he asked about hospitals that did work in this area, he was given the name of Gillette Children's Hospital. In the summer of 1972 he visited the brace shop at Gillette, and later he was invited to return for a more formal job interview.

The men in the brace shop had never quite fit into the life of the hospital, and Jean Conklin thought some changes were needed.

> We had three Swedish men.
> . . . They were excellent
> craftsmen, but they knew very
> little about administration.
> They didn't progress very well.
> They didn't keep up with
> the latest things, and some
> changes had to be made.

Dan Rowe, who worked in the brace shop for many years before starting his own company, described them as "saddle makers and luggage makers. They were excellent leather workers and did beautiful work." Marty Carlson understood why some of the nurses and physical therapists did not like working with the men in the brace shop: "Virtually all of them chewed snuff, and if they didn't chew snuff they smoked, and many of them did both. They were not a very refined lot."

Jean Conklin was impressed by Marty. He remembered the

interview in Dr. Winter's office, being asked why he wanted to change careers and how he would supervise employees. Jean Conklin's memory suggests that the decision to hire Marty was more spontaneous.

> He came in and I started
> asking him questions. I went
> down and got Bob Winter
> and he came and we both sat
> there and talked to him for
> more than an hour and a half.
> I said to Dr. Winter, "What do
> you think?" "Oh," he said,
> "grab him."

Marty was thirty-one when he became director of the brace shop in November 1972. He'd had no experience making braces or artificial limbs, and it took time for some of the older men in the shop to trust him. He relied on the skills of such people as Mike Pearl, Fran Hollerbach, Paul Quade, and Gene Berglund while he tried to convert the brace shop into an orthotics and prosthetics department. Jean Conklin and Bob Winter sent him to hospitals around the country so that he could learn from other facilities, and he studied

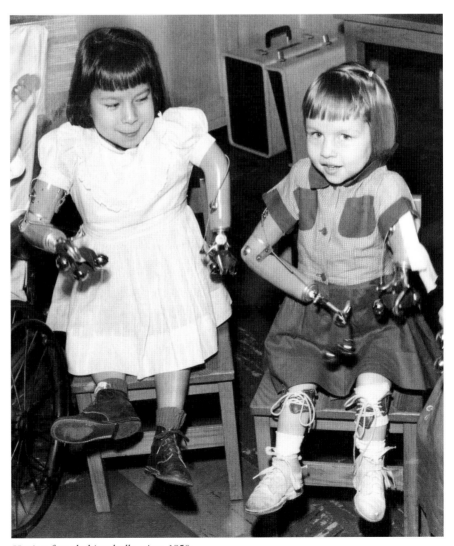

Having fun shaking bells, circa 1950

the practical aspects of using braces and artificial limbs by attending short courses at Northwestern University's medical school.

Marty quickly became involved in aspects of the hospital outside his department.

> My second morning on the job I attended something the nurses called "morning meeting" in which they went through about a dozen names of children who were of special concern. I remember thinking it was almost miraculous that I could go to work and be a part of the discussions about how to be helpful and possibly solve some of the problems and difficulties those children were up against.

His excitement was tempered by the discovery that medical decisions were made in a style very different from his previous work.

> I came to my position at Gillette from a background that was totally outside of medicine and health care. I was totally oblivious to the kind of hierarchical, almost caste-like system that tends to exist in medicine. I really think that if I had studied nursing or physical therapy, for instance, and been through an internship before coming to that position I would have been much less forward in my quest to learn. . . . I had come out of the physical sciences in which rigorous thinking was everything. Students questioned and challenged their professors or supervisors or anybody as long as they had a factual, scientific basis to support that question or challenge. I am so thankful for the many surgeons who tolerated me and evidently took my questions and my manner at face value.

Over the next decade the brace shop changed dramatically. Braces and artificial limbs were redesigned, and leather and buckles were replaced by thermoplastics and velcro. The staff was divided into working groups, and innovation was encouraged. New devices were created, such as seating arrangements for children who lacked the ability to sit and were poorly positioned in their wheelchairs.

Without being aware of it, Marty Carlson had arrived in the middle of profound changes at the hospital itself. The name he chose for the brace shop contained the essence of a new direction for the hospital: Habilitation Technology Laboratory (HTL). The polio epidemics had created an expectation that the work of the hospital was to restore children to their former health and activities, to "rehabilitate" them after their lives had been knocked off course by an unexpected event. But polio had disappeared, and other problems were more urgent: cerebral palsy, spina bifida, muscular dystrophy, and brain and spinal cord injuries. While many children with these conditions could participate in society, some could not and it became important for the hospital and its staff to help them and their families cope with their problems. Marty saw the work of his department as something more than producing braces and devices.

> I guess I have been impressed, as I look back over the many years of working with children with physical impairments, how the essence of successful habilitation is really connected more with the function of the mind and emotions than with the function of the body. The definition of successful habilitation, as it developed for me, is essentially to bring a child to the age of eighteen with an optimal degree of functional independence, an optimal degree of financial independence, and a constructive view of herself or himself in society.[17]

In a way, the hospital faced the same dilemma. It could not be "rehabilitated" or restored to the way it had done its work in the past. The era of long hospital stays and separation from family and friends was over. The hospital needed to rethink its own place in society and how it could help children in the future.

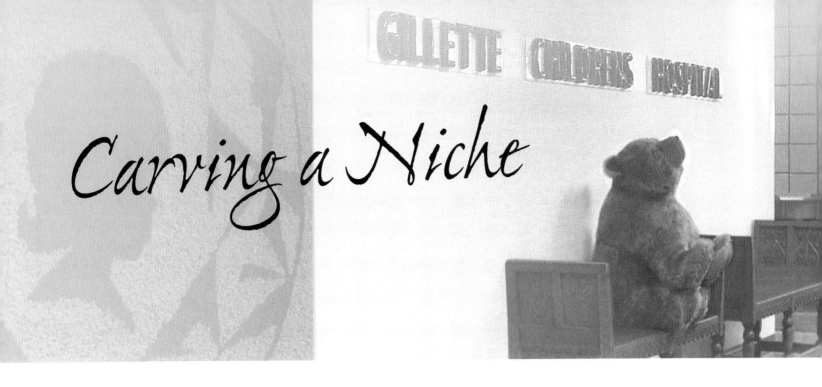

Carving a Niche

Until 1959 the children who received care at the hospital had one thing in common: they were poor and their families could not pay for health care. In 1959 the Minnesota legislature permitted the hospital to accept children from Minnesota whose parents had health insurance; at the same time the hospital was directed to bill their insurance companies for the cost of the child's care.

Most insurers disputed the state's right to collect insurance money since the hospital was operated by the state; individual families were not billed for their child's stay, and they were not expected to pay for costs not covered by insurance. The legislative action, which was intended to expand the hospital's services to more children with disabilities while reducing the cost to taxpayers, moved the hospital toward a different relationship with other hospitals and doctors.[1]

Although the effect on the medical community was small, the hospital was now a competitor for those children who had the money

to pay for their care. Other hospitals seemed unconcerned, but an action by the Gillette medical staff in August 1961 did not go unnoticed. At their monthly meeting a representative from the state attorney general's office discussed the possibility that the doctors also could charge insurance companies for their work. The minutes of the hospital's medical staff meeting on December 16, 1961, reveal the concern felt by some doctors in the community. A group of private surgeons appeared at the meeting to complain that the hospital was infringing on the private practice of medicine.[2]

Concerns about the hospital's future already were being expressed within state government. In November 1961 the Department of Public Welfare transferred the hospital to the new Division of Rehabilitation Services, directed by Leo Feider. After a year in his post, Feider asked permission to attend the medical staff meeting of February 2, 1963. He noted the steep drop in the number of new cases of poliomyelitis, and the increasing reports from field clinics sponsored by the state and attended by Gillette physicians that children with cerebral palsy had many unmet needs. He asked

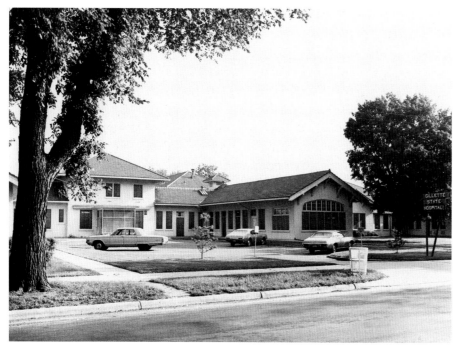

Gillette Children's Hospital, circa 1960

the medical staff whether it was time to decentralize the orthopaedic care of children by reducing the amount of care given at the hospital at Lake Phalen and expanding the number of clinics held at sites around the state. The medical staff thought field clinics were a poor use of their time since the Gillette doctors did little more than offer second opinions for children already receiving care close to their homes. The minutes suggest that the staff sensed that Feider's visit was not a casual one: "To some extent the medical staff is still confused as to why the meeting was necessary. They wonder if there are possible ideas of changing the present program of Gillette Hospital or of eliminating our program completely."[3]

By the summer of 1963 the staff had turned its attention to another matter. Chief of Staff John Moe felt that some of the staff physicians relied too heavily on the resident physicians and did not spend enough time with their patients. He brought this issue to the staff meeting of July 20 and suggested solutions. Moe had been in contact with Dr. Burr Curtis, medical director of Newington Children's Hospital

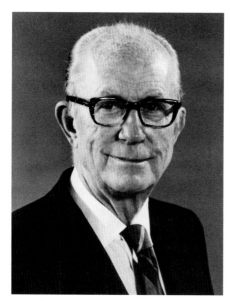

Dr. John Moe, circa 1970

near Hartford, Connecticut, and he felt that the Newington model of care might be appropriate for Gillette. Newington was an independent hospital that served children with many of the same problems seen at Gillette. Dr. Curtis supported the concept of organizing his hospital to meet all the needs of a child, not just the orthopaedic problems. Newington was one of the first hospitals to champion the idea of a "team approach" to children with disabilities. Dr. Moe suggested that Gillette study the Newington model. He also asked the staff to consider developing a rotation system under which each doctor would be responsible for a group of hospitalized children for three months at a time. The staff was skeptical, but agreed to invite Dr. Curtis to visit so they could hear more. They flatly rejected a rotation scheme and suggested instead a mentoring system in which the younger staff doctors worked with the older doctors until they had gained experience.

Dr. Curtis visited the hospital in January 1964 and described the Newington method in great detail. Apparently the medical staff was not convinced, for they chose to pursue the mentoring system they had suggested earlier. Many of the older staff physicians felt strongly that the hospital's trend towards clinics focused on a specific diagnosis or problem, as exemplified by the Spine Service, would lead to the development of physicians who knew a lot about a few things but lacked broad perspective and maturity. Dr. Cole and Dr. Harry

Hall were particularly vocal about this. They wanted to continue to see children with a broad range of problems. They wanted to decide if a child needed the expertise of another doctor rather than having a scheduling clerk direct the child to a specific clinic. The staff formalized the mentoring arrangement in February 1964. A group of the older, more experienced doctors was given senior attending staff status; the younger doctors were designated junior attending staff physicians and assigned to work directly under the supervision of a senior staff member. The senior staff included Drs. Wallace Cole, Carl Chatterton, John Moe, Harry Hall, Frank Babb, and Roland Neumann. The junior staff list included Drs. Robert Winter, Wayne Thompson, Thomas Comfort, Joe Tambornino, L. A. Nelson, and Edward and Elmer Salovich.

While not satisfied with all aspects of this arrangement, Dr. Moe recognized the strength of the older physicians and accepted the plan. From his own experience with children with spine deformities he knew the value of focusing on specific problems, and over the next two years the medical staff continued to discuss specialty clinics during their monthly meetings. Two distinct groups emerged from the discussions. One group continued to believe that specialty clinics would lead to the development of physicians who were not well-rounded. They also thought it unlikely that every condition seen at the hospital could have its own clinic. The other group thought that specialty clinics would lead to a better understanding of the children with those problems and would result in more consistent care. By late 1965 the specialty clinic group had won out. In January 1967 the hospital's clinic schedule was reorganized, with days of the week dedicated to specific problems. Monday became cerebral palsy day, Tuesday the day for hip and foot problems, Wednesday remained the day for spine problems, and Friday was for children who needed artificial limbs or had hand problems. Thursday was an open clinic day, allowing some of the doctors to continue to see children with a variety of problems.[4]

Meanwhile, Jean Conklin, who found much to like in the Newington model, took a step that was to lead to the hospital's move to a new site. In March 1965 she withdrew a portion of her biannual funding request from the legislature. Her original request had included $350,000 for a new outpatient department, but she had become convinced that the buildings at Phalen were so old and poorly organized that huge amounts of money would be needed to make the hospital more functional. She did not want to do a series of small projects that would never add up to an effective remodeling of the campus. Instead she asked the legislature to fund a study of the hospital's future. That request was honored and the firm of James Hamilton and Associates was hired to conduct the study. They began work in January 1966.[5]

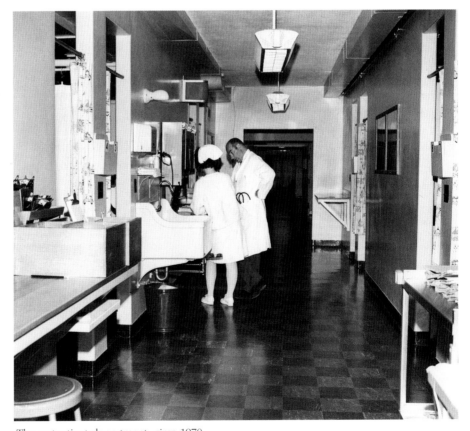

The outpatient department, circa 1970

The consultants quickly identified the key questions to be answered. Should children with disabilities receive care in specialty hospitals like Gillette, or should they receive that care in good general hospitals? Should taxes be used to support hospitals? Are public hospitals as efficient as private hospitals? Is there a difference between acute and chronic childhood illnesses? To what extent should the state support the cost of educating young doctors, nurses, and therapists? The question of state funding for the hospital was particularly pertinent. On January 1, 1966, Congress enacted Public Law 89–97, which initiated Medicare and contained a provision for children. Title XIX gave financial support to poor children with disabilities who were under the age of twenty-one so that they could receive comprehensive medical care. In the face of this federal program, the consultants wondered if Minnesota should continue as the only state with a children's hospital fully funded by tax dollars.

In August 1966 the consultants presented their conclusions: the hospital should continue to exist but should move from its campus at Lake Phalen to new quarters adjacent to an established medical center that could support its work. They recommended that the new facility be built to house between sixty and 100 children, and that admission be open to any child with a problem consistent with the usual work of the hospital. They also recommended that supervision of the hospital be transferred from the Department of Public Welfare to a hospital governing board appointed by the governor. And, they strongly recommended that the hospital become effective at billing insurance companies and Title XIX programs to offset legislative funding.[6]

Medical staff members were supportive, but concerned about portions of the recommendations. They wanted to make sure that the hospital would maintain its identity and continue to place strong emphasis on orthopaedic problems. In September 1966 a committee consisting of Drs. Thomas Comfort, Frank Babb, and John Moe was formed to summarize the opinions of the staff. Listing several reasons the hospital should continue to exist, the committee stated that medical expertise for difficult or unusual problems was hard to come by and would be lost if the hospital closed. This, in turn, would make it more difficult to educate young doctors. The committee described the value of specialized facilities and staff in the care of the children, with orthopaedic nurses and skilled therapists as examples, and pointed out that the hospital provided continuous care throughout childhood, which was important to families. The committee also supported the need for a new facility, for a full-time medical director, and for an effective system of state-sponsored field clinics throughout the state, in addition to the clinics held each day at the hospital.

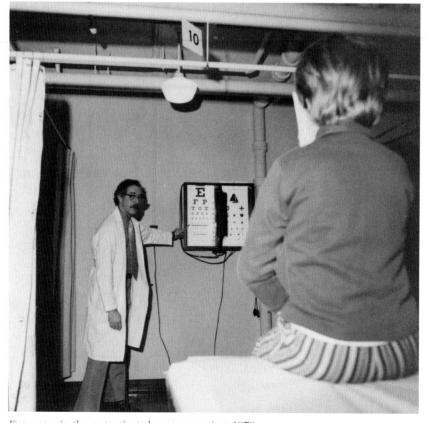

Eye exam in the outpatient department, circa 1970

The committee report was discussed in detail at the staff meeting on December 10, 1966, and strongly endorsed, with one important exception. Dr. Cole offered an amendment stating that the hospital should be rebuilt on the Phalen site. He was adamant that if the hospital moved away it would lose its identity and become lost within a larger medical complex. The depth of his feelings on this issue is captured in his plea to his colleagues: "Don't give up your birthright!" The staff adopted Dr. Cole's amendment and sent its report to Governor Harold Levander in February 1967 as a counterpoint to the Hamilton recommendations. As an addendum, they included a copy of the presentation Dr. Curtis of Newington Children's Hospital had made to the medical staff in January 1964. They stated that Gillette Children's should copy the Newington model.[7]

In early 1968 the question of the hospital's future came to the attention of the Welfare Subcommittee of the Senate Committee on Public Welfare, chaired by Senator William Kirchner. The committee reviewed the Hamilton study and asked Commissioner of Public Welfare Morris Hursh for additional information. In his response Hursh included a report by Jean Conklin and John Moe that charted the decline in polio and bone infections among the hospital's patients and showed how the hospital had become more effective in offsetting state financial support. By that time forty-eight percent of the patients had some form of private insurance;

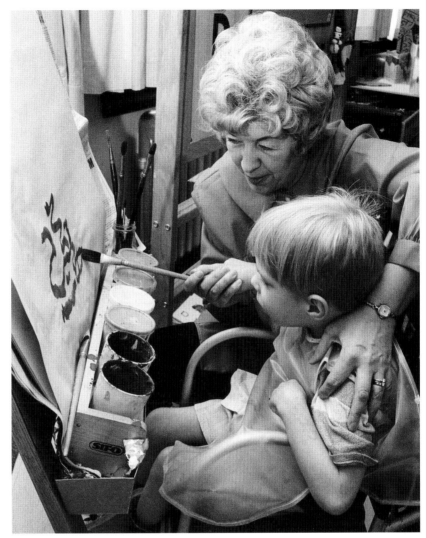

Painting, circa 1970

twenty-two percent qualified for the Title XIX federal program; eight percent paid for their own care; and only twenty-two percent relied entirely on the state for the cost of their care. Despite the position of the medical staff, Moe and Conklin recommended that the hospital move to a new location and specifically mentioned the campus of Fairview and St. Mary's Hospitals in Minneapolis and St. Paul-Ramsey Medical Center in St. Paul as possible sites. Their position was summarized in a single paragraph.

Now we are again confronted with the question of the need for a Gillette State Hospital and its location. We are strongly of the opinion that there is a need for such a hospital in our state for the total care of the handicapped child. We feel it should be relocated and that it must be orthopaedically oriented. The present facility does not lend itself to the most efficient program financially or medically. Its physical facility, in part, is consistently going to require more and more expensive remodeling. The hospital staff, very extensive in makeup, is not being used as efficiently as it could be because of the building's architectural style. And, the hospital is too small to offer the gamut of medical facilities required for complete diagnosis and care of the patients we are called upon to treat.

Senator Kirchner was troubled by the difference of opinion about the best site for the hospital. Representatives of a number of Twin Cities hospitals appeared before the committee to describe how Gillette Children's would function at their facility. Kirchner asked Jean Conklin and Dr. Robert Winter, now medical director of the hospital, what the children's parents preferred. Winter and Conklin sent a questionnaire to 2000 parents and received replies from 1100. They reported that while ninety-eight percent of the parents wanted the hospital to stay at Lake Phalen, ninety percent said they would continue to use the hospital if it moved to a new location. The parents also wanted the hospital to improve its outpatient area, expand its visiting hours, and improve communication between doctors and families. However, the Welfare Subcommittee declined to make any recommendations during that session of the legislature.

On October 27, 1969, Commissioner Hursh took a public stance on the issue of relocation. He recommended that the Lake Phalen site be closed and that the hospital be associated with another medical complex in the Twin Cities. The next day, the *St. Paul Pioneer Press* and the *Minneapolis Tribune* reported that the medical staff strongly disagreed with Hursh. The fight continued into the 1970 legislative session and finally was resolved in the Welfare Subcommittee, still chaired by Senator Kirchner. A motion by Senator Robert Brown of Stillwater to rebuild the hospital at Lake Phalen was defeated by a single vote, and was followed by a successful motion by Senator John Anderson of St. Paul to build a new facility, either at Lake Phalen or a site to be determined later. Although the location was uncertain, the decision meant that the hospital would continue as a distinct institution.

In 1971 Governor Wendell Anderson appointed a special legislative committee to consider where the hospital should be located. The committee was fortunate to be chaired by Clifford Retherford, who had worked in hospital administration for twenty-five years, including experience as chair of the board of Methodist Hospital in St. Louis Park, Minnesota, during a major construction project at that facility. Other

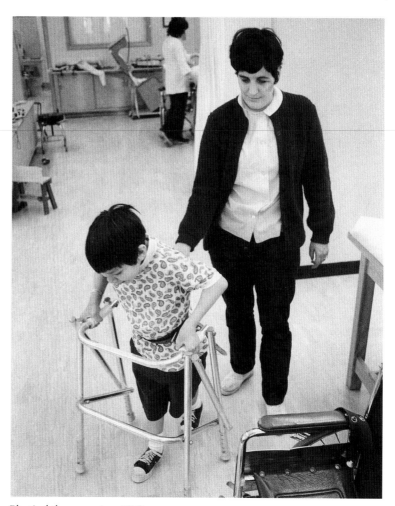

Physical therapy, circa 1970

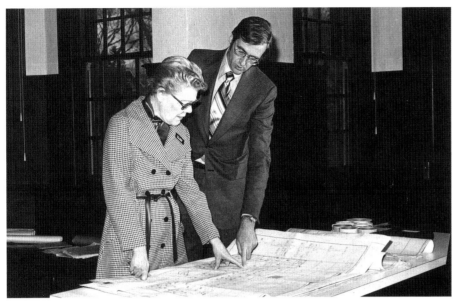

Jean Conklin and Dr. Winter, circa 1975

committee members included Dr. Ellen Fifer of the state Department of Health, Dr. Robert Winter, Dr. Richard Jones, an orthopaedic surgeon in the community, and citizens who did not have medical expertise.[8]

In December 1971 the committee sent letters to the major medical centers in the Twin Cities requesting proposals for moving Gillette Children's Hospital to one of their sites. A major restriction was placed on these proposals: the legislature expected the new Gillette to occupy up to sixty beds that would be made available by the hospital at the new site. On February 17 and 18, 1972, representatives of Children's Hospital of St. Paul, University Hospital, the new Minneapolis Children's Hospital (under construction at the time), and Minneapolis General Hospital (about to be rebuilt and renamed as Hennepin County Medical Center) outlined their proposals. Later that month,

St. Paul-Ramsey Medical Center and Fairview Hospital also presented their proposals.

Over the next several months revised proposals were received, and considerable political maneuvering was endured. In the end the requirement that the new Gillette make use of existing licensed hospital beds gave St. Paul-Ramsey Medical Center an advantage. Ramsey could give up sixty beds and was conveniently close to Lake Phalen. Children's Hospital of St. Paul was favored by some of the doctors but that hospital simply couldn't give up any of its beds. In fact, they were about to rebuild their own facility. A decision was made to move the hospital to St. Paul-Ramsey, an echo of the decision that had been made seventy-five years earlier when the hospital began its life at City and County Hospital in St. Paul.[9]

In 1973 the legislature acted on another Hamilton recommendation. The hospital was removed

from the control of the Department of Public Welfare and a not-for-profit corporation, known as Gillette Children's Hospital, was created with a board appointed by the governor. The board was required to make annual reports to the legislature and submit audited financial statements. Chaired by Cliff Retherford of the site search committee, the board took charge of the move to the St. Paul-Ramsey campus; $3.9 million was appropriated for new facilities and construction was started along University Avenue on the north side of the Ramsey campus. Patients and staff were transferred to the new hospital over the span of a week in April 1977.[10]

After the move the hospital's board asked Jean Conklin to visit county public health and welfare officials throughout the state to make certain they knew about the hospital's new location. She traveled 8,400 miles in six months and visited all but three counties. Then she resigned on December 16, 1977. Her assistant, Joseph

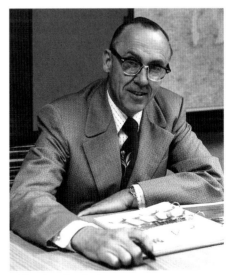

Clifford Retherford, 1977

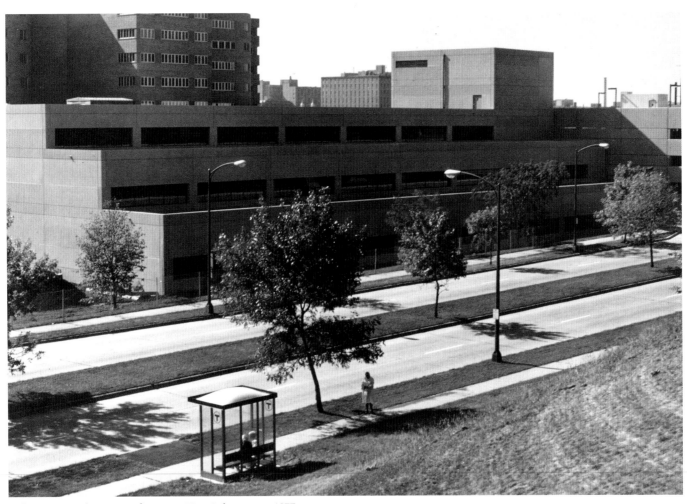

Gillette Hospital portion of Ramsey Hospital campus, 1977

Brown, succeeded her. In recognition of her twenty-eight years of leadership, Governor Rudy Perpich declared January 25, 1978, Jean Conklin Day throughout the state.[11]

Dr. Cole's 1966 prediction that a move would hurt the hospital's identity proved to be true. Despite Jean Conklin's efforts to inform county officials that the hospital was moving, not closing, referrals of children began to drop. The administration was overwhelmed with the transition to the new site and the work of balancing its budget without a state appropriation.

After a year of struggling with these problems, Joseph Brown resigned and was replaced by Norman Allan, a manager at St. Paul-Ramsey Medical Center. In 1980 Dr. Robert Winter resigned as medical director after finding that his private medical practice did not allow him enough time for his administrative tasks at the hospital. A less obvious but equally damaging change occurred in the medical staff. The system of senior and junior attending staff physicians did not survive the move to Ramsey, and many of the doctors lost their sense of commitment to the hospital. Some of

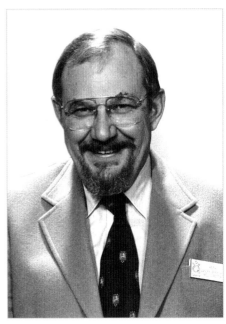

Dr. Keith Vanden Brink, 1980

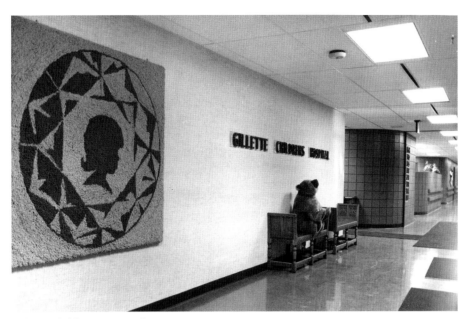

Gillette Children's Hospital, 1977

them simply could not afford to donate one or two days of service to the hospital each week. At the same time, the expectations of children's families changed. They demanded a more direct relationship with the same doctor at each clinic visit or hospital stay. The changes in the medical staff made this difficult, and family physicians and pediatricians did not know which doctor would be seeing the children they referred to the hospital.[12]

The new medical director was Dr. Keith Vanden Brink, a native of Iowa who was a pediatric orthopaedic surgeon at the Campbell Clinic in Memphis, Tennessee. Dr. Vanden Brink took the position on a full-time basis in 1980. His daily presence and friendly manner made him attractive to patients and their families, and to pediatricians and family doctors in the community. While physicians who came to the hospital part-time saw their work load

decreasing, Dr. Vanden Brink quickly became very busy. The growth of his practice demonstrated that the community needed the services of the hospital and its doctors, but some members of the medical staff felt threatened

by Dr. Vanden Brink's success.

By 1986 budget deficits forced the hospital board to take dramatic steps. In February 1986 the hospital placed a moratorium on hiring, and later that year the staff was reduced by twenty percent. The following August, Dr. Vanden Brink left Gillette to work at the Shriners Hospital in Lexington, Kentucky, and Dr. Robert Winter was asked to assume his old post. The board had come to believe that the hospital could not survive without both new management and an affiliation with one of the children's hospitals in the Twin Cities. In late 1986 the board signed an agreement under which Minneapolis Children's Medical Center would provide key administrative support. When Norman Allan resigned as administrator, Patricia Klauck, president of Minneapolis

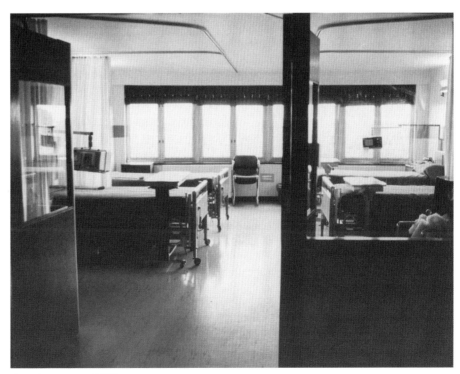

A patient room, 1977

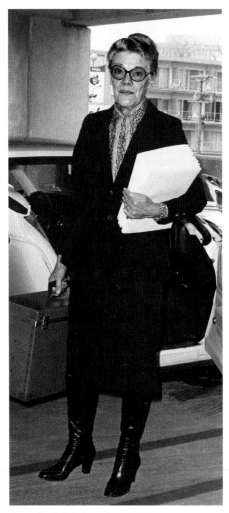

Jean Conklin's last day, 1977

Children's, appointed Margaret Perryman, a member of the administrative staff at Minneapolis Children's, to become the chief operating officer at Gillette.[13]

Margaret Perryman was born in Wyoming in 1947 and grew up in Nebraska and Montana. She graduated from Carroll College in Helena, Montana, with a degree in medical technology. After working in laboratories in children's hospitals in Los Angeles, Denver, and Portland, she became the first laboratory manager at Minneapolis Children's Hospital. While working there she earned a degree in

business administration and this, combined with her administrative experience, made her a good candidate for the job at Gillette. Many, however, assumed that Gillette's management contract with Minneapolis Children's was a prelude to a merger, and Perryman told Patricia Klauck that she was concerned about that perception.

> I told her that if she wanted
> me to downsize the organiza-
> tion and prepare it to be trans-
> ferred over to Minneapolis
> Children's, then she shouldn't
> hire me to do the job because
> I wouldn't do that very well.
> If she wanted the organization
> to grow and expand and capi-
> talize on opportunities, I told
> her I would then take the job
> because that's what I would
> do well. She told me that in
> order for a tree to grow it
> might need to be pruned. I
> agreed but I told her I didn't
> want to be a mortician for the
> organization. It was only
> because she assured me that
> she wanted the organization to
> grow and flourish that I agreed
> to take the job.

Despite acting as an advocate Margaret Perryman knew nothing about the hospital. "When I arrived at Gillette," she recalled, "I was astonished that, while I had worked in pediatric healthcare in the Twin Cities for fifteen years, I really didn't know what Gillette did." In her first year she laid out the steps the hospital would have to take: help the employees and doctors believe the hospital's

recovery was possible; reduce costs; and improve the reimbursement the hospital received for its services. She found one asset already in place. In spite of the financial problems, employees and the medical staff all believed they were doing important work.[14]

In 1988 a legislative measure cut the hospital's last ties to state government. Gillette Children's Hospital, now an independent organization, became a member of Minneapolis ChildCare, the parent organization of Minneapolis Children's Medical Center. At first Minneapolis Children's was not interested in a merger because of concerns that Gillette would be a financial drain on a merged

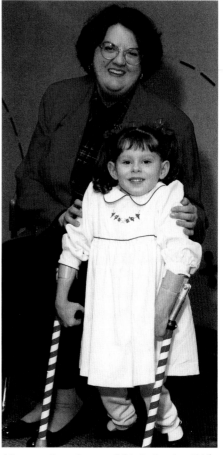

Margaret Perryman and Maria Steele, 1996

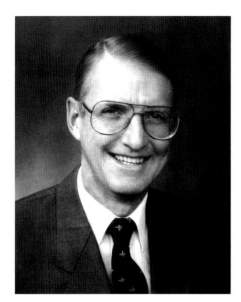

Dr. James Gage, 1995

organization. The reluctance to pursue a merger proved to be a blessing for Gillette. Under Margaret Perryman's supervision the hospital quickly stabilized its finances, and with the leadership of Dr. James Gage the medical staff and the programs of the hospital took on new structure. Dr. Gage, a native Minnesotan, had been a member of the Gillette medical staff in the 1970s before becoming a full-time pediatric orthopaedic surgeon at Newington Children's Hospital in 1976. He had developed a strong interest in children with complex orthopaedic problems and had helped Newington develop a premier motion analysis laboratory to study the walking problems of children with cerebral palsy. He had helped Gillette build its own motion analysis laboratory in 1987, and was keenly interested in the survival of his old hospital. He returned to Gillette in 1990 as medical director.[15]

As Minneapolis Children's turned its attention to building

more space for its patients the idea of a merger with Gillette became more attractive. A merger would bring all of Gillette's activity to the Minneapolis Children's campus and would make the costs of construction more manageable. The Gillette board members saw the merger in a different light. They were convinced that children with orthopaedic and neurologic disabilities were a unique group who needed a hospital fully focused on their needs. Rather than seeing a merger as an opportunity to improve this mission, the board feared that Gillette's work would not receive the priority it deserved. The board of Minneapolis ChildCare, now the parent of both organizations, listened to arguments from both sides. They decided not to merge the two hospitals and took the additional remarkable step of releasing Gillette Children's from its relationship with ChildCare. Gillette was free to pursue its own mission,

much stronger because of the new management style it had inherited from Minneapolis Children's.[16]

In the early 1990s Gillette remained concerned that its St. Paul-Ramsey Medical Center facilities were too small to support growth. Gillette had organized its work into six major areas: children with orthopaedic problems, cerebral palsy, spina bifida, brain or spinal cord injury, epilepsy, and children with severe lung and neurologic problems who required constant support from breathing machines. An emphasis was placed on everyday problems that did not require surgical treatment. This work was directed by Dr. Linda Krach, a pediatric physiatrist. Later programs for children with arthritis and children with chronic pain would be added. Discussions were opened with Children's Hospital of St. Paul about relocating Gillette to new facilities next to that hospital. It was thought that Children's might

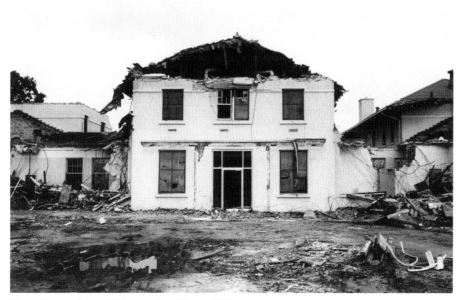

Demolition of the old hospital building, 1980

be a better partner for Gillette's work than Ramsey, and that an opportunity to build there might allow Gillette to solve some of its space problems. In the end Children's Hospital of St. Paul found merger discussions with Minneapolis Children's to be a higher priority and the negotiations with Gillette stopped. Margaret Perryman's feelings after all of these merger conversations were shared by many at Gillette.

This was perhaps a case of divine intervention. We were cruising down a path which would have likely resulted in a merger [with St. Paul Children's] and a gradual loss of mission, and we weren't aware that there was danger ahead. I think too many of us were listening too much to critics who labeled Gillette as isolationist and uncooperative, and we were trying to demonstrate to those critics and to ourselves that this was not the case. This was a golden opportunity for Gillette. With Minneapolis and St. Paul engaged in merger discussions [there was an] opportunity for Gillette to solidify [its own] future. We had chased a relationship with each of the other children's hospitals thinking they were the answer and, in truth, we probably had the answer all along. Each time we walked away from affiliation discussions the organization's mission became clearer and the staff's resolve to succeed in its mission became more emphatic. Gillette was now fully ready and convinced that it was possible to remain independent.

With merger discussions behind it the hospital focused on its programs with the assumption that it would remain located next to St. Paul-Ramsey Medical Center, which was renamed Regions Hospital in 1997. A new generation of physicians emerged to take responsibility for the care of the children referred to the hospital and its clinics. Between 1987 and 1995 the total number of children coming to the clinic for care increased from 11,015 to 14,031 annually; the number of surgeries performed increased from 586 to 1,106, and the number of children admitted for inpatient care increased from 797 to 1,035. The average hospital stay for inpatients dropped to six days in 1997. The transition from a state institution to a private facility that could serve all children in the state was complete.

After the move to the St. Paul-Ramsey campus, all but one of the buildings at the old hospital site on Ivy Avenue near Lake Phalen were demolished. Only the Michael Dowling building, opened in 1925, was spared, but it quickly fell into disrepair and remained unoccupied for several years as no one found a use for it. The land reverted to the city of St. Paul, which boarded up the building against vandalism. It became a stopping place for the homeless, and was damaged by a fire. A number of organizations considered occupying the building, including a church and a community theater, but those plans fell through because of the condition of the building and the cost of remodeling. Only the efforts of a group of neighborhood residents and former patients known as the Gillette Heritage Association kept the Dowling building from being demolished. Finally, in 1993, the Minnesota Humanities Commission took possession and spent more than two million dollars to create a conference and educational center for teachers. The dream of Jessie Haskins and Arthur Gillette to provide education for the hospital's young patients continued in a place where those children once had gathered to learn.[17]

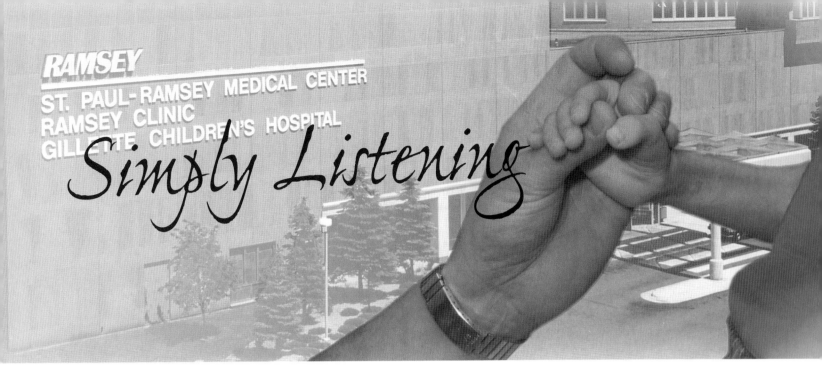

Simply Listening

After the hospital moved from Lake Phalen into downtown St. Paul there was no dominant disease or disorder to capture the attention of the public. As in the days of tuberculosis and polio, children continued to come to Gillette to be treated for deformities of bones and joints that were present at birth or appeared later due to injuries or abnormal growth.

Those problems, however, had not increased in frequency. Instead, more care was focused on children whose problems had not received as much attention. Their diagnoses included cerebral palsy, spina bifida, muscular dystrophy, brain and spinal cord injury, and childhood arthritis. Sometimes the diagnosis was established before the child ever came to Gillette; for other children Gillette was the place where answers were found. By focusing on children with orthopaedic and neurologic causes of disability, Gillette became a resource for other hospitals and doctors.

Children with isolated problems and those with extensive problems both found a very different hospital than the one encountered by those who had gone to Lake Phalen. For the newcomers, most of their treatment came during visits with their doctors in the outpatient department, with hospital admissions less common and quite brief. By 1997 the average hospital stay for a child was only six days. In response to the needs of the children the medical staff expanded to include more medical specialists than just orthopaedic surgeons. These changes meant lots of travel for

families and numerous visits to the outpatient department for evaluations by a variety of doctors, therapists, and experts in braces and equipment designed to make daily life easier.

In the early decades of its existence the hospital provided nearly all of the treatment needed by a child. After the move from Lake Phalen that was no longer true. Orthopaedic surgeons practicing out in the community treated some of the problems previously seen at Gillette, and it became more common for Gillette's physicians to see children with severe, complicated, or unusual problems.

Many of the children with conditions like cerebral palsy and spina bifida already had received care from other physicians and hospitals before they came to Gillette for treatment. In those cases physicians, therapists, and other workers at Gillette Children's became partners with their colleagues out in the community in providing care for the children and their families. The stories of these children and their parents show how lives can be changed by a disability, and they also show how Gillette has helped children today.[1]

Molly O'Rourke was a typical seven-year-old from St. Paul when she fell at a swimming pool.

A friend of mine called me up and asked me if I would like to join her and her mother and go swimming with them. Who would have known that one day at the pool would result in almost ten years of pain? That summer day at the pool is very hard to remember. I remember it as a very confusing, scary, and most of all, painful day.

Molly had broken her hip and needed surgery. She was hospitalized at Children's Hospital of St. Paul, where she received good care from Dr. Paul Yellin and the staff. However, the fracture had disturbed the blood flow to a part of Molly's hip. This meant that she needed to wear a brace to protect her hip while it healed. Like most children, Molly did not like her brace.

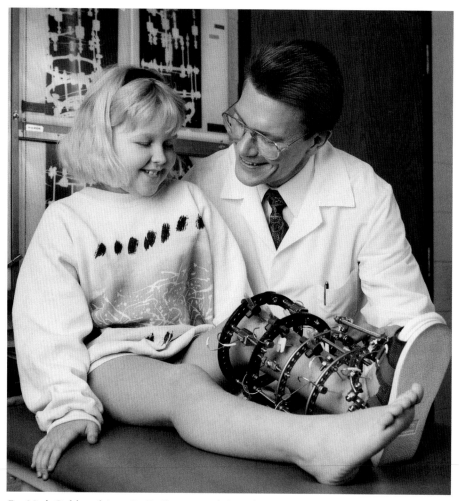

Dr. Mark Dahl and Amy Jo Freiburger with her Ilizarov fixator, 1991

When I first got my brace I didn't want to wear it. I felt like an alien. I noticed everyone's eyes on me whenever I went out. I would hear comments like "Mom, what's on her legs?" or "She looks different!" "Different." I hated that word! I just wanted to be like everyone else. All my classmates would make fun of me and no one understood why I had this brace.

Dr. Yellin visited Molly's school and explained the brace to her classmates, which made life easier but didn't make the problem go away. In some ways, it drew more attention to it.

All my teachers felt sorry for me and I soon learned to hate sympathy. I didn't like everyone fussing over me and I still feel that way. As I look back and think about how my life was so different from most kids it still makes me sad. I always thought my hip problems would just be temporary and some day I would be a "normal" kid.

Mary Kay O'Rourke, Molly's mother, measured the ways that

life changed for the rest of the family.

Simple things like buying clothes she could wear with the brace and walking through metal detectors which would go off were new considerations for us. Molly was worried about fitting through doorways and getting on the school bus. I remember in particular a family vacation in Washington, D.C., the summer she had her brace on. Washington probably was not the best choice but it was an opportunity to join my husband on a military trip. There was far too much walking involved with seeing the various monuments, and I also remember Molly setting off the metal detectors at the Federal Bureau of Investigation Building. I was appalled when they frisked her, as it was very obvious the leg brace had set off the detector. It became apparent to me then that we needed to even change the way we planned our family vacations.

Molly's hip improved somewhat, but the pain returned and her doctor sent her to Gillette with the hope that she might find help there for this difficult problem.

I was devastated when I found out I would need to have another surgery but I knew I needed to do something to help ease the pain. I was afraid, though, that it would be second grade all over again: another ruined summer! The surgery and crutches, it wasn't that bad and my hip was feeling pretty good. To my surprise the pain came back. When I started to use a cane I was really embarrassed. When I walked into school I never heard so many comments and so many people talk about a piece of wood! I just wanted to scream "I HAVE A BAD HIP!" I soon got really sick of telling my story to the world.

Molly's recognition that there was no cure for her problem was followed by sadness. Mary Kay O'Rourke described her own struggle to help Molly through the hard times.

I believe part of the change was a result of being in a new school and having new friends who didn't understand how she could be in such pain or why she couldn't keep up with them. . . . The pain she experienced forced her to come home early from dances and other social activities with her friends. She would also get upset with her friends for not understanding why she needed to go home. As a teenage girl Molly is concerned with her appearance and her acceptance by her peers. I believe that her limp and the

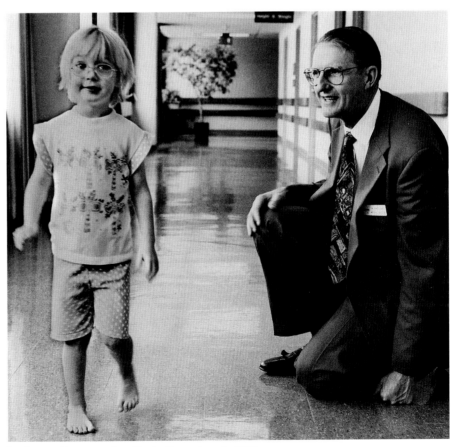

Dr. James Gage watches Linda Rogers's gait, 1992

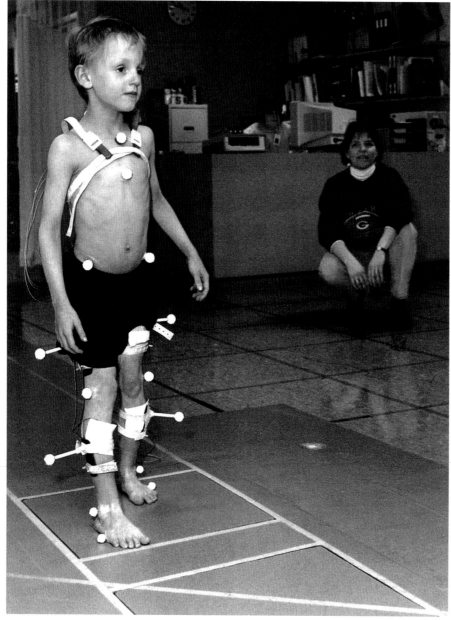

Zachary Gale in the Gait Analysis Laboratory, 1997

replaced with weaker fibrous bone. After surgeries at Gillette, Katie's pain improved but did not disappear. Terry Blummer was pleased that his daughter felt better but was very aware that her problems had not gone away.

> Don't get the impression everything has been perfect. We still are frustrated at the inability to diagnose all of Katie's pain problems. We deal with this every day at home and it causes us to worry about what it could be. Lately we met as a family with [one of Katie's doctors] and she thinks stress has something to do with Katie's pain. Talk about tough decisions! Do we stop parenting the way we have for eighteen years because it might cause some stress? I think we have raised a great kid and our parenting has something to do with that. On the other hand, Katie has suffered enough and I would do anything to stop her pain.

Dina Blummer, Katie's mother, shared these worries.

use of crutches and a cane have contributed to her having a poor self image. I can tell her she is a beautiful and talented young lady but it doesn't matter. As a mother I find these years very frustrating. It is difficult to know she is not only experiencing physical pain but also emotional pain as a result of her disability.[2]

The O'Rourke family was not alone. Katie Blummer of Cottage Grove grew up with pain in her legs, and many years went by before the cause was discovered. When she developed severe pain in her hip she was sent to Gillette, where she was found to have fibrous dysplasia, an uncommon benign condition in which the usual strong bone of children is

> Our daughter's condition seems so hard to "fix." I worry about the future. Will she continue to experience daily pain? Will her condition continue to worsen? Will she be able to function away from home at college next year? Will she lead a normal adult life? How will her mental wellness be if she is in pain?

The problems of a child with cerebral palsy are just as unexpected and surprising as those of injury or illness, but the outcomes often are different. When a child breaks a bone or is sick parents assume that the injury will heal or the illness will go away. Although the event is unexpected and worrisome the best response is patience because things will improve and life will return to normal. Conditions like cerebral palsy are different. The problems are more complicated and never ending. Life is dramatically changed, as the stories of several families demonstrate.

Cerebral palsy is the most common childhood condition that results in lifelong disability. Three or four of every thousand children have cerebral palsy, which is defined as a disorder that reduces the brain's ability to control the behavior of muscles. The event that changes the function of the brain occurs during pregnancy, near the time of birth, or early in childhood. There are many causes, including malformations of the brain, ruptures of blood vessels in the brain, injuries, and infections, but the most common problem associated with cerebral palsy is premature birth. The earlier a child is born and the lower the birth weight, the higher the risk that the brain will not function normally and cerebral palsy will occur. Children with cerebral palsy are as diverse as any other group of children. Some have minor problems with using an arm or a leg but are able to do all the things other children can do. Others are profoundly disabled, with severe

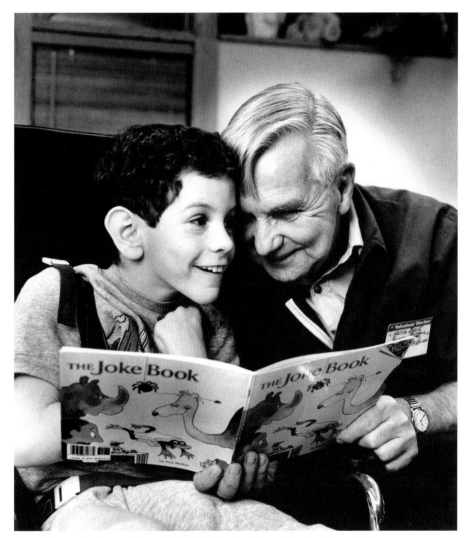

Evan Flam enjoying a joke with Merle Bjork, a hospital volunteer, 1991

spasticity, mental impairment, and deformities of their arms, legs, and spine. Many children with severe cerebral palsy are completely dependent on their family for the most basic things in life.

By the time most children with cerebral palsy come to Gillette for treatment, their parents have gone through very difficult experiences. For the staff at Gillette, listening to those experiences is the first step toward understanding the hopes of parents. Lynn and Scott Rodby of Elk River were parents of three

children under four years of age when Lynn became pregnant with twins. Although the pregnancy was a surprise they were excited. It was a difficult pregnancy that included three admissions to the hospital to prevent premature labor. Finally, twin boys, Robert and Steven, were born five weeks early by Caesarean section. The boys each weighed more than five pounds, and they were expected to do well after a stay in the newborn intensive care unit of a hospital in the Twin Cities. Lynn remembers what happened next.

On the fourth morning after the twins' birth I was preparing to be discharged from the hospital when the phone rang. It was the nursery calling to say that something was wrong with Steven. They believed that he had suffered a massive brain hemorrhage and were conducting tests to determine the extent. Could I please call my husband and have him come down to the hospital as they would like to talk with us?

The news was not good.

At the meeting we were told that the results of the tests did indeed show that Steven had suffered a severe intraventricular hemorrhage. In lay terms he had severe damage to both halves of his brain. The pressure from the bleeding caused the blood to invade the brain tissue, causing irreversible damage. In short, nothing could be done for him. When we asked what his life would be like we were told that he would be severely mentally and physically handicapped. He would have no reasoning or cognitive abilities. He would be deaf and blind. He would not have the ability to enjoy life as we knew it. In fact, he would not even have the ability to know us. We were devastated.

Many parents share this feeling of being helpless. Sometimes

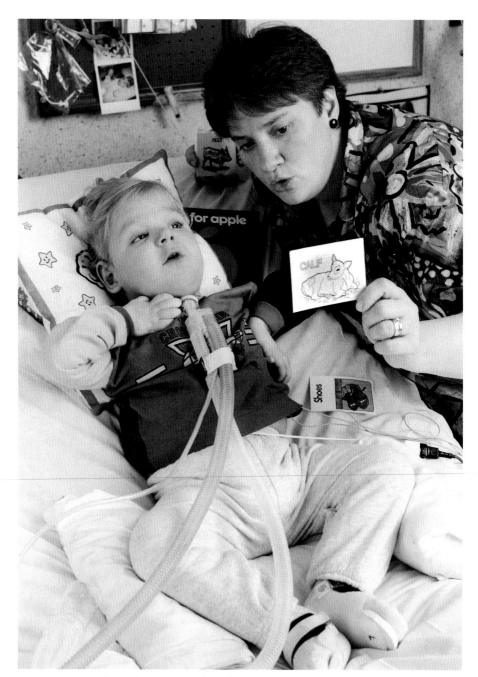

Peter Braun gets bedside schooling from Debra Zenker, 1994

the news is so overwhelming that parents find it hard to accomplish even simple tasks. Marian Bonkowske of Princeton felt that way after her son Brad was injured at age three.

I am the mother of a sixteen-year-old severely handicapped child. Our son suffered a traumatic brain injury almost thirteen years ago. There are many events in the first couple of weeks of his hospitalization that I don't remember. I guess my body was still in a state of shock but I do remember meeting with the doctor when he told us he thought our son was going to survive but that it was going to be a long road to recovery. Up to that point I dreaded each meeting with the doctor because I was afraid he would be asking us to make that dreaded decision of whether or not to turn off the machines. There was such a rush of relief at that point that nothing else in the world mattered. Our young son had fought to survive and he would fight to recover. As a family those first four or five months were lived on the proverbial roller coaster.

Shock often is followed by the hope that there was a mistake or that things would turn out better than expected. Lee Lemke was three months old when he nearly died from sudden infant death syndrome (SIDS), sometimes called "crib death." Annette Lemke, also from Princeton, remembers the first days when her son was in the intensive care unit of a hospital in Minneapolis.

It was the first day, actually the first two days, and Lee's dad and I went into the hospital chapel. I remember both of us praying out loud and telling God to take Lee's arm, to take Lee's legs, but don't take his mind when in fact we knew very well that that was the one thing that had been taken. You know, there is always that little bit

of hope because such miraculous things happen with children.

Cheryl and James Brandes of Crystal shared that hope for their daughter Ellen, who was born in California.

Our first response after Ellen's birth was to pray that she would live. We had no clue about how serious her handicap would be or the dramatic change in our lives her birth would bring. Ellen's first month brought seizures, renal failure, and eating problems.

We didn't yet realize she would also be afflicted with cerebral palsy, microcephaly, and mental retardation. In retrospect maybe it's a good thing we didn't know how severe her problems were. We might have given up. Instead we lived day to day waiting for everything to eventually be all right.

But the problems never go away and parents find that they must commit a large part of their lives to the special needs of their child. At a hospital like Gillette Children's the treatment of a child

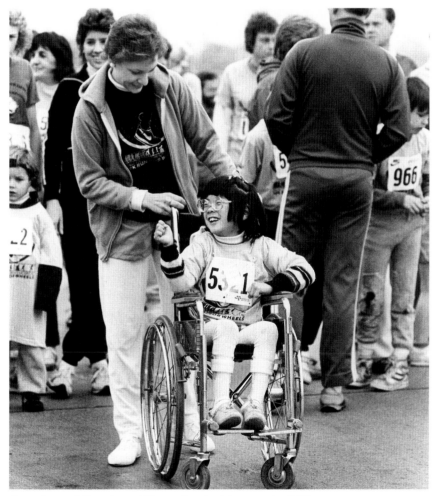

Race day and Bonnie and Poppy Sundquist are ready, 1985

with a serious disability requires an awareness of the struggles of their parents and family members. The health problems of a child with a serious disability affect marriages and other children in the family. Annette Lemke described what happened to her family.

Lee really challenged my husband's and my relationship. I don't remember the two-and-a-half years that Lee lived at home. He required twenty-four-hour care and he was on an apnea monitor [to make sure he was breathing] which would sometimes go off twenty times a night. I do not remember our other two children. I don't remember anything that may have been real important to them or something that might have happened to them. I do remember that it was like two families living under one roof. My husband took care of the girls and I took care of Lee.

Parents become isolated and lonely, and they fear what other people think about them and their child. Annette Lemke found it difficult to take Lee places.

Encountering society was especially scary for me at first. I remember the first time that I was going to take Lee [out in] public in his wheelchair and being so very frightened. I was afraid of what people would say or do. The very first time that I did this we went to McDonald's and I had my niece along with me. She was probably sixteen at the time and was a wonderful girl who was definitely blessed with a lot of love and talent for dealing with special needs people. On that day we stopped and I sat in the car and said, "I'm not sure I'm ready for this." I remember her saying, "Well, no time is a good time like the present." So with her courage we took Lee and the wheelchair out and wheeled him in and got our food and sat down. This wonderful child's voice said, "Look mom, look at that neat stroller!" The mother tried to shush the child but I knew at that point that it was my cue to inform the child about Lee. It was from that point on that I decided that Lee would be a learning tool of sorts for people in society.

Sometimes it is best for a child and parents if the daily problems are shared by other people. Stress can bring people to the point where they simply can't

Cody Warne with his mother Becky and Paula Vander Shaaf, 1995 handle it anymore. Then they have to ask for help. That happened to Annette Lemke.

We decided to place Lee in a foster home after I realized that I was becoming sick mentally and physically. This was the most trying time of our lives, dealing with the county. We made several attempts to get some type of financial help. I had insurance through my work but that insurance only paid sixty dollars a month for respite care. We needed more than that. So we asked the county if they could help us in that area. Their reply was that you either quit your jobs and become totally dependent and receive all the benefits or you get none. And to us that was not an option. It was ludicrous and absurd. We continued to try and take care of Lee without respite care until I realized there wasn't much time left. I was unsure of whether I would cross the line, which was very scary to me and to my husband. It was frightening not knowing whether your next move was going to be sane or insane. We finally went to the county for the last time and said this is it, we are asking you to find a foster home soon. At this point I was unsure of what would happen. I was suicidal and I was unsure if I would cross that line or take someone else's life. It was very frightening. I never want

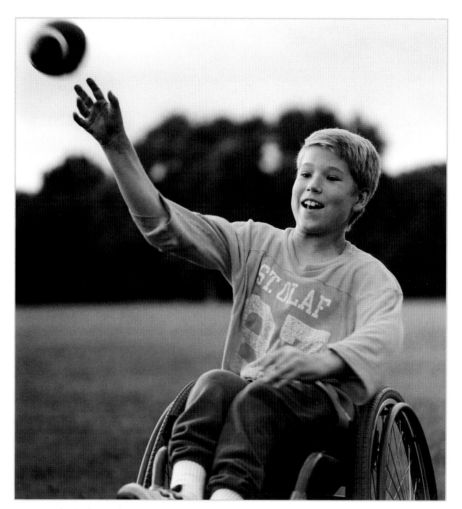

Jeremy Thiel shows his passing style, 1993

to experience anything like that again.

Most parents do not find it easy to ask for help caring for their child. The Lemke family was divided about foster care. Annette Lemke described the feelings of the family.

The placement was very hard on my husband and our youngest daughter, but easy on me and our oldest daughter. I had given our oldest daughter a lot of responsibility from the time she was five years old, asking her to sit in

the house for an hour and listen to the heart monitor so I could just go outside. That was a lot of responsibility for a five-year-old.

Marian Bonkowske felt pushed to make a decision to place Brad in foster care.

The decision for foster care placement was a very agonizing decision. A lot of thought went into it but we were almost forced into making the decision by a threat from our insurance company to discontinue hospital payments. They wanted our son placed in a long term care facility over a hundred miles from our home. That is when I learned very quickly to become an aggressive person, which is not really in my personality at all.

Some people believe that foster parents take in children simply because they are paid to care for them. The Rodbys had a positive experience with two retired nurses who helped take care of Steven for more than a year, but they had a poor experience with a second foster home.

The Lemkes and Bonkowskes had good feelings about Kathy and Steve Orton, foster parents for Lee and Brad who live in the Orton home except for a few days each month when they are with their parents. Marian Bonkowske described it this way.

> Our son's foster parents are truly sent from heaven. Mrs. Orton and I are so in tune with each other I sometimes think in our former lives we were sisters. We even look somewhat alike. Right from the start I did not have any doubt about the welfare of our son living [with] and being cared for by someone else. I am very involved in every area of our son's life and consulted about everything.

Foster parents can become very close to the children in their home, and that brings challenges. Kathy Orton described the feelings of a committed foster mother.

> One thing I really had problems with at first was the bond between the parents and the child. It was so strong! I just couldn't figure it out because we were the ones that were taking care of him and doing everything for him and yet that bond was still there no matter how mentally or physically handicapped the child was. . . . Brad's and Lee's parents have been just really supportive of us and have been really good and these have just been little hurdles. It is important for them to feel like they are really a part of everything that we do although we are doing the actual twenty-four hour work. The support they give us is so important and we don't want to do anything to mess up the bond between the child and the parents. It is really important for these kids and I can't say enough about that. It was hard for me at first but as time has gone on it has gotten easier. I have realized the kids need all the support and bonding wherever they can get it.

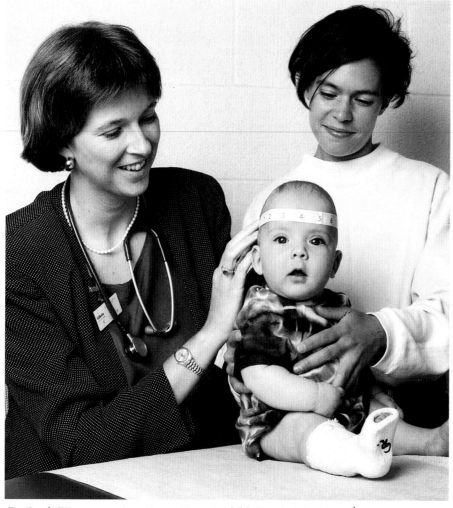

Dr. Sarah Winter examines Karen Urman's child, Danzig (Ziggy) Norberg, 1993

Being foster parents is not for everybody. The Ortons have found it to be challenging.

Most couples would not be able to do the work we do. We are together constantly! We really have very little time together alone but we work together. Sometimes it's kind of tricky. Like this: "Okay, this is your department, you're going to handle that, and this is my department." Sometimes you have to do each other's work, and that gets interesting. We have learned a lot.

Parents of children with severe disabilities have good and bad experiences with medical workers. Lynn Rodby remembers feeling powerless, particularly right after Steven's brain hemorrhage and while he was still in the newborn intensive care unit.

After much tearful discussion with Scott that night we went back to the hospital and informed the doctor that we wanted Steven taken off the respirator. We had assumed in our ignorance that we had the authority to do this as his parents. The hospital told us that they had a mandatory seventy-two-hour waiting period and if at the end of that time the EEG test showed no brain activity he would be taken off. If Steven survived the waiting period, his prognosis remained the same. We were very upset, as we defi-

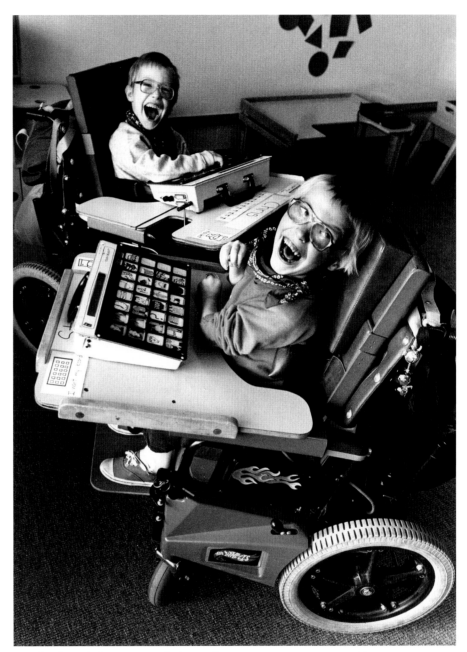

Touch-talkers help Steven and Christopher Majetic communicate, 1989

nitely did not want to see one of our children live that way. We felt that if Steven was taken off the respirator and survived on his own, then that was what God wanted. If he did not survive then that also was what God wanted. We wanted Steven, we loved him, he was our child, and

we felt it was our responsibility to decide for him and to take care of him.

Although that event happened before Steven received care at Gillette, every survey of parents of children treated at Gillette has confirmed the importance parents place on being

151

included in important medical decisions for their child. Parents also dislike the assumption that they are not capable of understanding medical information. Marian Bonkowske described her frustration with some of the behavior she encountered among doctors and nurses.

In the medical profession as well as in everyday business encounters there are many wonderful people but there are also a few jerks. I have not found a guidebook to teach us how to deal with them but in our situation we had to learn very quickly. The most frustrating part of the problem is the attitude of some of the doctors that since I have a handicapped child I must have a lower IQ than the norm. There is a big difference between explaining things in layman's terms and being talked down to. Like having the attitude that since I wouldn't understand anyway why take the time to explain things to me. We have found this not only true in the medical profession but also in dealing with social services, school administrators, insurance companies, and home health care agencies. There is a stigma in our society that anyone using the welfare system, in our case medical assistance, is an uneducated and second class citizen.

Sometimes one person can make all the difference. Cheryl Brandes felt that way about one of Ellen's doctors, a pediatrician who went out of his way to help them.

We were lucky we met Dr. Jeffrey Alexander during a frequent clinic visit. Ellen had chronic ear infections and unexplained high fevers so we spent many hours in clinics. He was a wonderful man with a true affection for special needs children. He introduced us to the Cerebral Palsy Center preschool and Gillette Children's Hospital. He truly saved our lives and our marriage.

Former patients who as children received care at Gillette Children's Hospital, before its move to the Ramsey campus, remember people from their long hospital stays. Those long hospitalizations are rare now, and parents and children remember the people they encounter during their visits to the outpatient department. Annette Lemke appreciated seeing familiar faces: "One of the nicest things about Gillette is that after nine years we still get to see the same faces, which is a wonderful feeling. It is a feeling of friendship and those friends greet us every time we come to Gillette. It is your receptionist sitting at a desk and always smiling, always greeting, always making that first impression."

Like all parents, the parents of severely disabled children wonder what place their child will find in society. They are all too familiar with the whispering they hear around them: A disabled child has problems that take time and energy away from other people. It costs a lot. Is it worth it? These problems aren't going to go away. This child is very retarded. I can't understand him and he can't take care of himself. He'll never contribute anything. What kind of a life is this? Yet these parents have forged a truce between their hopes and reality, and they are seeking practical solutions to everyday problems they face. Most have found purpose in the lives of their children. Kathy Orton described the effect Brad Bonkowske had on his special education classroom.

Brad is in a special needs class and there are some kids in there who really have a difficult time reading, especially reading aloud to a teacher or a classmate. They just can't do it. But, they love to read to Brad. This is one of Brad's jobs at school. He goes into a room with another special needs child who has difficulty reading and that child will read to Brad when they would not read to anyone else. Brad never complains about their reading. He gets excited and he loves it when they read to him. It has just been a really good experience.

Kathy Orton remembered that Lee Lemke had a similar effect on a child in his class.

When Lee was in fourth or fifth grade there was a little

girl that they didn't know what to do with because she was so introverted. She would never answer a question in class, and she sat there with her head down most of the time. For some reason she really took to Lee and she started getting interested in his care, what they did with him, what was right and what was the wrong thing to be doing with him. She started talking to other kids about it, things like "Lee's hands need to be here" or "We need to push Lee's head up because he's drooling." Pretty soon she was becoming more extroverted in other classroom things and started answering questions. The teacher could not believe how this child had blossomed over the year and she really believed that it had everything to do with Lee.

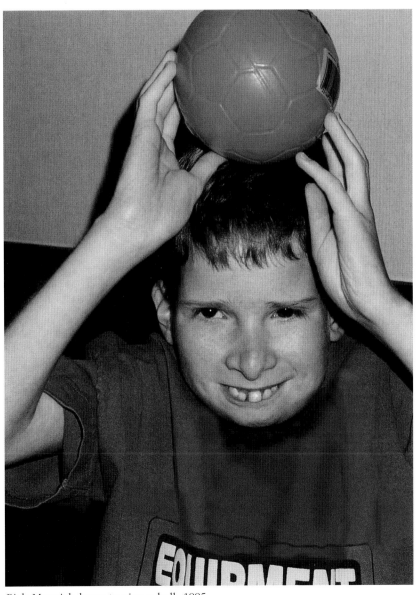

Rick Muenich loves tossing a ball, 1995

Life with children with disabilities also has its lighter moments. Like other children, they are able to surprise their parents. Freddie Poole of St. Paul has spina bifida, a condition in which his spine formed abnormally before he was born. His legs are paralyzed, so he goes places in his powered wheelchair. He had watched the public buses that stopped at the corner near his house, and one day, when he was ten years old, he went on a great and unplanned adventure. He rode onto a wheelchair accessible bus and went sightseeing. An alert bus driver noticed that Freddie didn't seem to have a plan, and when he radioed his dispatcher he found out that Freddie's mother and the police were frantically searching for him. When Freddie got home, he got hugs, and he was grounded.[3]

Cheryl Brandes speaks for every parent of a child with a long-term disability:

"Our biggest fears concerning a mentally and physically disabled child are concerns about changes in state aid and medical coverage. Also, what if something happens to us? Who will care for Ellen? Where will she live? Who will keep her safe?"

As the twentieth century closes some parents have a new dilemma. Instead of choosing between methods of treatment they now can choose whether to have a child with a disability, for some conditions are detectable before a child is born. The matter of choice confronted Terry and Karen Goken.

My husband and I went in for a twenty week ultrasound at our regular hospital, and after looking the baby over and congratulating us and telling us everything was fine they asked if we wanted to see anything else on the screen. I said I wanted to see his hands. Then the room got very quiet and we were sent to our doctor who told us that there might be some problems with our baby's forearm and a couple of digits on his hands. The next day we had a level two ultrasound. At that ultrasound we found that our baby had nothing below either elbow and that one of his thigh bones was half the length of his right. This was an incredible shock. We were not prepared for this, and we were also asked at that time if we would like to terminate the pregnancy because they talked about the quality of life this little guy would have.

The Gokens wanted as much information as possible.

We wanted to talk to a specialist right away to see what our son's life would be like, how we could try to prepare for this, and what corrections could be done. So we went to Gillette and were seen within the week. I can't tell you what a relief that was. Here are two parents carrying news they never expected to hear and searching for answers and any piece of the puzzle. It was just nice to go and confer with the doctor and see what he thought this was going to be like for our son. I remember that visit clearly. There were a lot of tears as he explained the ultrasound, and a lot of hope. I gained hope thinking that even though surgically they couldn't just go in and put two arms on him and make everything better it was going to be okay, that there was a place for children to learn to deal with what they had in a very positive atmosphere.

The Gokens made up a list of the positives and negatives for their son, hoping that the arithmetic would make their decision easier. In the end, for them, the arithmetic didn't matter, and they chose to finish the pregnancy. Their son was born with the deformities of his arms and legs that had been predicted. Was the ultrasound and the turmoil it brought worthwhile? Karen Goken believes it was.

It has been a different situation but I am also glad I found out while I was pregnant. It gave us a chance to get over the initial surprise, regroup, think about what we wanted to do and how we wanted to handle everything. We got excited again about our son's birth! I can't imagine finding out at delivery.

Karen Goken identified the fear that overwhelms parents, and described what helped her.

I think the best advice I could give anybody would be that usually we are just scared when we find out this news because we have never dealt with it. It is just ignorance. The more that my husband and I read, the more people we talked to, the less we were scared. Then we kept the focus on our son. If you can keep in mind that this is your child and there is nothing you wouldn't do for this child, then there is hope and you just learn what you need to do to get the job done.

For a hundred years, children and their parents have confronted their fears at Gillette and have searched for ways to cope with life. They have learned from others, sometimes doctors and nurses and therapists. More often they have learned from each other, meeting on the ground of common experience, sharing the treasure, and the challenge, of serving another person in need.

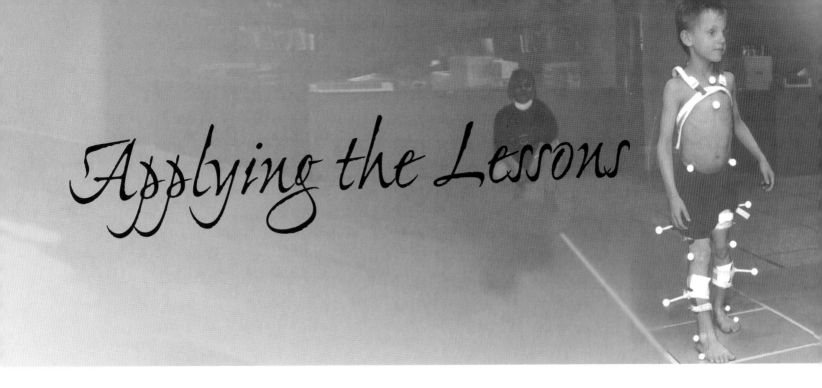

Applying the Lessons

The ancient Romans thought the deity Janus presided over beginnings and endings, and they commonly placed his image, a man with two faces looking in opposite directions, over doorways. We name the first month of our calendar year after him, a time when we look back on our experiences while looking forward to a new start. We must end this book in the same way.

If we do not consider what the past means for the future, then the history of Jessie Haskins and Arthur Gillette and those who came after them will be little more than a timeline and a recitation of sterile facts.

One person with a good idea can make a difference.

Jessie Haskins showed us that a good idea can take root and grow, just like the proverbial mustard seed yields a great tree. She understood poor children, for she grew up in a single parent family and watched her mother struggle to make ends meet. She also under-stood children with physical dis-abilities, having grown up with severe scoliosis and then carried the additional burden of a badly broken shoulder. And Jessie understood the feelings of parents who could not help their children as much as they might like. We can imagine the conversations she had with her mother when the family made another move, or when she could not return to Carleton College after her two years in the academy there, or when there was no money to treat her scoliosis.

When Jessie listened to the visitor from St. Paul during late 1895, and heard the story of a homeless disabled child, her reac-tion was simple: something must be done for children like this. She pursued this by talking to her friends and her professors, and came to the conclusion that the best way to help such children was to educate them and give them the same medical care available to other children. That concept was so fundamentally fair and just that it ultimately persuaded the representatives of the people of Minnesota to create the nation's first state-supported hospital for children with disabilities. A centu-ry later, more than fifty thousand

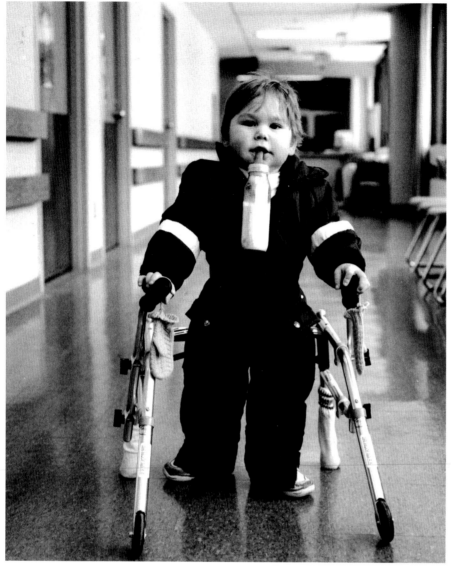

Timothy Klein, 1993

children have received care at that hospital. Jessie Haskins showed us that one person can make a difference.

Our notion of disability is changing.

The commitment of the legislature in 1897 was not completely altruistic. While the legislators were sympathetic to Jessie Haskins, they were suspicious of Arthur Gillette's motives. He won them over when he pledged to provide free care and when he pointed out that healthy children might grow up to be self-supporting and tax-paying citizens. As a result, for many years the hospital's annual reports mentioned the number of children who were cured or improved.

Arthur Gillette, Stephen Mahoney, and Elizabeth McGregor knew that the state expected to see a return for its tax dollars. Children who were not expected to improve often did not receive treatment, the most obvious example being those children with significant mental impairment. It would be unfair to portray the legislators or hospital staff of that time as uniquely insensitive to these children. Society itself shunned the mentally incompetent, and children and adults with these problems often were sent to state institutions. While the improvement in an individual child's life was important, the state estimated the worth of its investment in disabled children by calculating the contributions those children might make to society as adults. By that reckoning, it made little sense to invest in a child who could not be expected to contribute. The polio epidemics tended to reinforce the notion of investing in children who could be expected to recover their health and become self-supporting adults.

Poliomyelitis did more than create fear among parents and dominate the work of Gillette Children's Hospital for two generations. It also defined the American notion of how people become disabled and how they should be helped. Polio epidemics were sudden, indiscriminate, and overwhelming. One day children were doing the common things of life and the next day they were helpless. It did not seem to matter whether their parents were rich or poor, or where they lived. Polio went where it liked and seemed almost wanton in its behavior. One child might have weakness in an arm or a leg while the next child was paralyzed and fighting just to breathe. And none of the thousands of children who filled up hospitals could be blamed for what had happened to them. They were victims. The average citizen had a reason to identify with polio victims: their child might be next. The polio virus was a common enemy to be hunted down and eradicated. With enough money and research, a vaccine was found and other children were spared. Children with polio were easy to understand and support. They were the heroes of the war, struggling to get back to a normal life.

Since the end of the polio epidemics, society has been faced with children whose disabilities don't fit this model. Today, in addition to children who have an isolated physical problem that can be repaired or much improved, Gillette treats children with very complicated conditions such as cerebral palsy, spina bifida, muscular dystrophy, brain and spinal cord injury, and many others. In comparison to polio, many of these children are never "normal." Something goes wrong before they are born or early in their lives, and they never follow the usual development of a child. Often it is not possible to identify a clear cause for their problems, or something that can be changed or reversed. Some of the children are mentally impaired, and some always will need the help of others to accomplish the most basic daily activities. Many will need substantial medical care throughout their lives.

This picture is quite different from the child making a heroic recovery from polio. People whose lives have not been affected by a child with a complicated lifelong disability find it difficult to understand the needs of those children or the feelings of their families. There also is a tendency to place blame for the child's problems on someone else: a doctor must have made a mistake, the parents must have been incompetent, the mother must have done something wrong when she was pregnant. And today's budget-conscious society asks tough questions. What kind of care should be given to children who can't be cured? How much money should be allocated for children who can't join mainstream society? How much help do their families deserve? After a century, the tension between the needs of the individual child and the cost to the rest of society still is present.

Children with disabilities need a health care system that focuses on their problems.

Before 1920 the average child spent more than four hundred days at Gillette being treated for their problems. By 1950 this had been reduced to one hundred days, still long compared to the average stay of six days in 1997. Today people often view those long admissions as cruel. In fact, they were essential.

Before World War II most physicians were general practitioners, and most of their patients were adults. Physicians were just beginning to specialize in the medical care of children, the diseases and disorders that resulted in childhood disabilities were poorly understood, and there were no pediatric hospitals in Minnesota until the 1920s. Children received treatment in separate wards in adult hospitals, and even if a physician wanted to treat a child with scoliosis, clubfoot, tuberculosis, or polio, there were few nurses, therapists, and bracemakers skilled in treating those problems.

Transportation also was a major factor in the long stays at Gillette Children's Hospital. Until World War II, travel from rural Minnesota to St. Paul was chiefly by train, and most families could not afford such a trip more than once or twice in a year. Even when travel by automobile became more practical, a trip to St. Paul was still time-consuming and expensive. Most families had other children to care for, and it was hard to take the time from work or find someone to do the farm chores. Although separating children from their families was undesirable, the lack of expert medical care in local communities for the special problems of childhood disabilities, combined with the difficulties of travel, made long stays at Gillette Children's a necessity.

There were many good things about gathering the children into one place. They had a clean, safe place to live and they were given clothes and good food. They stayed as long as was needed to make them as whole as possible, and their parents did not receive a bill. No longer were the children oddities: they were with other children who shared their problems. They received an education, and they taught the doctors, nurses, and therapists about their diseases and disorders, thereby ensuring that the children who came after them were given even better treatment.

The first twenty-five years of the hospital were dominated by infections of bones and joints, especially tuberculosis. The next forty years were dominated by the problems of poliomyelitis. The hospital campus was large, with numerous wards and buildings, because children received their treatment as inpatients and because they stayed at the hospital for such a long time. The problems of travel now have been overcome, and much of the treatment the children need today can be given during visits to clinics held in the outpatient department, or during hospital admissions that last only a few days. This means the hospital, whose name became Gillette Children's Specialty Healthcare in 1997, is much smaller and less obvious in the community.

Gillette clearly has moved into a third phase in its existence. The conditions that bring children to a hospital like Gillette are uncommon, but together they comprise a group far larger than those with polio during the epidemic years. Between two and four of every one thousand children will be found to have cerebral palsy; and spina bifida, muscular dystrophy, and childhood brain and spinal cord injuries are even less common. Perhaps one child in a thousand is born with a clubfoot or a dislocated hip. Scoliosis, one of the more common problems of childhood, develops in two or three of every one hundred children, but only one child in a thousand develops a serious curvature. The rarity of these problems means that most community physicians, including pediatricians, family doctors, and orthopaedic surgeons, still do not feel comfortable treating a child with one of these diagnoses. Children with orthopaedic and neurologic disabilities still need health professionals who understand their problems and hospitals dedicated to their special needs.

Ten years ago, when hospitals were being closed and mergers were rampant, no informed health care economist would have predicted that in 1997 the last independent hospital in the Twin Cities metropolitan area would be Gillette Children's, the smallest and most specialized of all the hospitals. But will there be room for Gillette in a medical marketplace dominated by insurance companies and managed care organizations? Will those systems, so focused on adults and on common health problems, recognize the needs of children with uncommon disabilities? For one hundred years Gillette has focused on the needs of children with neurologic or orthopaedic health problems, and the hospital has gathered together doctors, nurses, therapists, and technicians who choose to dedicate their work to the needs of these children. Will children with disabilities have access to this care?

Medicine is more than a business.

Today the monthly meetings of the boards of directors of hospitals, insurance companies, and managed care organizations are filled with statistical reports that portray the health of the organization. Attention is focused on the numbers of patients, surgeries, and clinic visits. There is anguish over the amount of accounts receivable, the rate of bill collections, and the operating margins being generated. Discussion often turns to talk of mergers, strategic alliances, and political initiatives. What is harder to measure are the experiences of the children and families being served, and the people who serve them.

For more than fifteen hundred years, the Rule of St. Benedict has been a guide for men and women who choose to live in monastic communities. The Rule begins with simple advice: "Listen carefully, . . . incline the ear of your heart."[1] That is good advice for anyone who works at a place like Gillette Children's and encounters children whose lives have been changed by illness, injury, and deformity. The hopes and fears of children and their families may vary when they come to Gillette, but they have something in common: they need someone to listen to their story.

The stories of the past one hundred years teach us a most enduring lesson: medicine is measured by how lives are changed and improved. At its best, the business of medicine is transformational, not transactional.

Notes

GCSH Gillette Children's Hospital Papers, Gillette Children's Specialty Healthcare, St. Paul, Minnesota

GHP Gillette Hospital Papers, State Archives, Minnesota Historical Society, St. Paul, Minnesota

CCA Carleton College Archives, Northfield, Minnesota

MHS Minnesota Historical Society, St. Paul, Minnesota

MSA Minnesota State Archives, Minnesota Historical Society, St. Paul, Minnesota

MSLL Minnesota State Law Library, St. Paul, Minnesota

POA Pediatric Orthopaedic Associates, Historical Research Collection, St. Paul, Minnesota

UMA University of Minnesota Archives, Minneapolis, Minnesota

Orthopedics and orthopaedics are interchangeable terms used to describe the work of physicians who specialize in problems of the bones, joints and muscles. The official titles of professional groups favor the spelling "orthopaedic." The author has chosen to use this spelling throughout the book.

Some readers may be concerned about the use of first names, last names, or professional titles when referring to specific individuals in the book.

First names were used when the subject preferred to be identified in that manner, or when research indicated a first name was commonly employed (i.e. Miss Elizabeth for Elizabeth McGregor).

CHAPTER 1: PASSION AND EXPERIENCE

1. Letter from Carrie Haskins Backus to Elizabeth McGregor, February 20, 1946, including a biography of Jessie Haskins written by Ella Haskins Holly, (circa 1930), GCSH.

2. Reverend Delavan L. Leonard, *The History of Carleton College. Its Origin and Growth Environment and Builders* (Chicago: Fleming H. Revell Company, 1904); Leal A. Headley and Merrill E. Jardrow, *Carleton. The First Century* (Northfield: North Central Pub. Co., 1966).

3. Carleton College Faculty Records, March, 1895-1901, CCA; Young Men's Christian Association, "The Bible Work of the Young Men's Christian Association, 1895-6," Minneapolis, CCA; Carleton College, "President Strong's Report, June 14, 1897," CCA. This document demonstrates the strong social content of the Carleton curriculum. "The Junior and Senior classes have united during the past term in the study of Ethics. Special emphasis has been laid upon the subject of social ethics . . . includes a series of six lectures . . . by Reverend H. H. Hart of St. Paul, Secretary of the Board of Charities and Corrections, upon the work of the State in moral reform."

4. "State Board of Corrections and Charities," *Minnesota Executive Documents*, Vol. II (1900): 289–290, MSLL.

5. Jessie A. Haskins "An Institution for Deformed and Crippled Children," *The Minnesota Bulletin of Corrections and Charities* 38 (1896): 6–7, MSA.

6. Hiram David Haskins, family bible record of marriages, births, deaths, and letters, 1851–1887. Patchin-Patchen Family Papers, Special Collections Division, Northwest Room, Spokane Public Library, Washington.

7. Jessie Haskins biography.

8. Ibid.

9. Patchen papers.

10. Baldwin English and Classical Seminary (brochure), MHS. Backus was superintendent of the seminary that later merged with other schools into Macalester College.

11. Mrs. Backus' School for Girls (later named Oak Hill School) located at 489 Holly Avenue, St. Paul. Various brochures and student papers in Manuscripts Collection, MHS; Virginia Brainard Kunz, *Saint Paul: The First 150 Years* (St. Paul: The Saint Paul Foundation, Inc., 1991), 71.

12. *Annual Catalogue of the Officers and Students of Carleton College,* (Northfield: The Adams Press), 1883–84, 1895–96, 1897, 1898, 1899, CCA.

13. Michael John Dowling and Jennie Leonharda Bordewich, Dowling Papers, Manuscripts Collection, MHS; Lowell E. Jepson, "A Career Without A Parallel," *The Alumni Magazine* Vol. II (1) (1911): 1–12, CCA.

14. Jessie Haskins biography; United States Census Bureau, 1892, Kettle Falls, Washington, Eastern Washington Genealogical Society.

15. Student Records and Ledgers, 1893–1899, CCA.

16. Gamma Delta Society of Carleton College, *Recording Secretary's Book*, 1895–98, CCA; Gamma Delta Membership Roster, 1917, CCA. Jessie Haskins is listed as an alumna employed as an assistant city librarian, 2309 Illinois Avenue, Spokane, Washington.

17. Jessie Haskins, "The Need of an Institution for Crippled and Deformed Children," *Proceedings of the Fifth Minnesota State Conference of Charities and Corrections held at Red Wing*, 1896, (St. Paul: The Pioneer Press Company, 1897) 46–48, MHS; A. H. Pearson, "Altruism and Reform," ibid., 16–10, MSA. The agenda of this conference demonstrates the close link between Pearson and Hastings Hart.

18. *The Daily Pioneer* (St. Paul), November 19, 1896; *The Minneapolis Journal*, November 20, 1896; *The Daily Republican*

(Red Wing), November 16, 17, 18, 19, 1896, MHS.

19. *Proceedings Fifth Conference*, 1896, 46–48; "Dr. Hastings H. Hart, Secretary of the Board of Corrections and Charities, had listened to Miss Haskins' plea before the board in 1896 and had also become active in working for the project." Wallace H. Cole, *The Story of Gillette Children's Hospital, St. Paul, Minnesota*, 1972, GCSH; Carl C. Chatterton, "Gillette State Hospital for Crippled and Deformed Children," *Minnesota Medicine* 14 (1931): 439–440, GCSH.

20. J.A.A. Burnquist, "Arthur J. Gillette, M.D.," *Minnesota and its People*, Vol. IV (The S. J. Clark Publishing Company, 1924), 26–27, MHS; Idem, "Medicine and Dentistry," Vol. II, 1924, 107–128; Emil Geist, "Dr. Arthur J. Gillette—An Appreciation" *The Journal-Lancet* Vol. 4 (1921): 202–203, Boeckmann Library, St. Paul; "Dr. Gillette: surgeon and hospital-builder," *History of St. Joseph's Hospital 1853–1978*, (St. Paul: Communications Department, 1979), 17, St. Joseph's Hospital Archives; Leonard G. Wilson, "The Hospital for Crippled Children," *Medical Revolution in Minnesota: A History of the University of Minnesota Medical School* (St. Paul: Midewiwin Press, 1989) 89–92. Wilson provides an invaluable outline of the development of numerous medical schools in Minneapolis and St. Paul before the creation of the University of Minnesota Medical School; Catalogue of Hamline University for the years 1880–81, 1882–83 (Minneapolis: Johnson, Smith & Harrison, 1881), Hamline University Archives; Newton M. Shaffer, M.D., "The Care of Crippled and Deformed Children," in *Proceedings of the Twenty-Fifth National Conference of Charities, 1898*, (no publishing information), MHS. Shaffer discusses philanthropic efforts to provide orthopaedic care and training for handicapped children on the East coast and well as efforts world-wide.

21. Jane M. Hult, "Dr. Arthur J. Gillette and the Hospital for Crippled Children" (paper delivered at University of Minnesota History of Medicine Lecture, Gillette Children's Hospital, St. Paul, January 1986), GCSH.

22. A. B. Stewart, "Orthopedic Surgery as Applied in the Use of the Tenotome," *Northwestern Medical and Surgical Journal* 1 (1871): 349–359, GCSH.

23. Carl C. Chatterton, "Early Orthopedic Surgery in Minnesota," *Minnesota Medicine* 36 (1953): 360–363, GCSH; Leonard G. Wilson, "James E. Moore: Founder of Graduate Medical Education at Minnesota," *Minnesota Medical Foundation Bulletin*, GCSH; Wilson, *Medical Revolution*, 1989.

24. A sampling of Dr. Gillette's work and involvement in the medical community can be found in the many articles GCSH retains: "Bowed Leg. Combined Osteotomy and Osteoclasis," *Northwestern Lancet* Vol. 1 (1890): 121–122; "The Simplest and Most Rational Treatment of Club Foot" (paper presented before the Minnesota Academy of Medicine, November 1, 1890), *Northwestern Lancet* Vol. 1 (1890): 395–399; "Rachitis and Resulting Deformities" (paper read before Ramsey County Medical Society, May 26, 1890), *Northwestern Lancet* Vol. 1 (1890): 179–182; "Orthopedic Surgery As A Specialty" (paper read before Minnesota Valley Medical Society, December 1891), *Northwestern Lancet* Vol. 1 (1892): 50–54; "Pott's Disease With Special Reference to Treatment in the Upper Dorsal and Cervical Regions" (paper read before Department of Surgery of the Minnesota State Medical Society, June 17, 1892), *Northwestern Lancet* Vol. 1 (1892): 321–325; "Two Cases of Tuberculous Knee Joint Disease" (paper read before the Pathological Section of Ramsey County Medical Society, December 10, 1892), *Northwestern Lancet* Vol. 1 (1892): 128–129; "Mechanical and Forcible Straightening of Old Deformities of the Knee Joint" (paper read before the Section of Surgery of the Minnesota State Medical Society), *Northwestern Lancet* Vol. 1 (1895): 421–425; "Sprains" (an address delivered before the Ramsey County Medical Society January 25, 1897), *Northwestern Lancet* Vol. 1 (1897): 161–167; "Traumatic Spondylitis" (paper read before the American Orthopaedic Society, Washington, D. C., May 1897), *Northwestern Lancet* Vol. 1 (1897): 391–393; "The Duty of the State to its Indigent Cripple Children" in *Proceedings of the Sixth Minnesota State Conference of Charities and Corrections*, November 3–5, 1897 (St. Cloud: The Pioneer Press Co., 1898), 72–76, MSA; "The State Care of Indigent, Crippled and Deformed Children," *Proceedings of the National Conference of Charities and Correction*, June 15–22, 1904, Portland (Maine: Press of Fred J. Heer), 285–293, MHS; Board of Control, *Annual Report of the Board of Control, City and County Hospital for the Year Ending 1893* (St. Paul: St. Paul Herald Printing Co.), 1894, Ramsey County Papers, MHS; idem, 1894–96, (St. Paul: The Pioneer Press Co.). The annual reports at city and county record Dr. Gillette as the only orthopaedic surgeon for many years.

25. Hult, *Dr. Arthur Gillette*, 1986.

26. "Minnesota Good to Her Suffering Children. How Crippled or Deformed Little Ones Whose Parents Can't Afford to Pay Are Given the Best Medical Treatment," *Minneapolis Journal*, August 6, 1898, GCSH.

27. *House Journal*, 30th Sess., State of Minnesota, H.F. No. 749, pp. 498, 812–13, 842, 847, 858, 1101, 1114–17, 1167–68, MSLL; *Senate Journal*, 30th Sess., State of Minnesota, H.F. No. 749, pp. 891, 916, 921, MSLL.

28. "State Home for Cripples. How a Girl is Lobbying in Behalf of Children," *Saint Paul Pioneer Press*, April 7, 1897, MHS; "A Commendable Bill. State Home for Crippled and Deformed Children. The Work of a Carleton Girl for this Neglected Class," *The Independent* (Northfield), April 15, 1897, MHS; "Carleton News," *Northfield News*, April 10, 1897, MHS.

29. Jessie Haskins biography.

30. *Minneapolis Journal*, August 6, 1898.

31. Ibid.

32. *House and Senate Journals*, 1897.

33. *Minneapolis Journal*, August 6, 1898.

CHAPTER TWO: THE FIRST OF ITS KIND

1. University of Minnesota, Board of Regents, Minutes, August 25, 1897, UMA; *Minneapolis Journal*, August 6, 1898.

2. "News and Notes" in *The Charities Review* Vol. VII, September-February 1897–98, 796–798, MHS; Physician correspondence, GCSH.

3. *Laws of Minnesota for the year 1897*, Chapter 289, H.F. No. 749, MSLL.

4. University of Minnesota, Board of Regents, *First Annual Report of State Hospital for Crippled and Deformed Children* (Minneapolis: Rice Bros. Printing Co., 1898), 3–12, GHP; Board of Regents, Minutes, 1897.

5. Board of Control of St. Paul and Ramsey County, *Annual Report of the Board of Control, City and County Hospital for the Year Ending December 31, 1897,* (St. Paul: The Pioneer Press Co., 1898), 20, Ramsey County Papers, MSA; Letter from Ramsey Board of Control to Hon. D. M. Sullivan, Auditor of Ramsey County, July 9, 1897, Ramsey County Papers, MSA. The letter contains a detailed budget for maintaining City and County Hospital for 1898.

6. Board of Regents, Minutes, April 12, 1898; "Regents Meet," *The University of Minnesota Ariel* XXI (1898): 373, UMA. Contains announcements of faculty promotions.

7. *Minneapolis Journal,* August 6, 1898.

8. Board of Regents, Minutes, December 14, 1897; Arthur Gillette, M.D., "Annual Report of the Surgeon-in-Chief," in *Annual Report of the Board of Control, City and County Hospital for the Year Ending December 31, 1898,* 69–79.

9. Letter from Royal J. Gray to Elizabeth McGregor, January 14, 1920, GCSH.

10. Arthur Gillette, M.D., "Annual Report of the Surgeon-in-Chief," *First Annual Report of State Hospital for Crippled and Deformed Children,* 3–16.

11. "Biographical Sketches," *University of Minnesota Ariel* Vol. XX (1896), UMA, includes a biography of Honorable Stephen Mahoney.

12. Board of Regents, minutes, October 5, 1905, Physician's Correspondence, GCSH.

13. Arthur Gillette, M.D. "The Duty of the State to its Indigent Cripple Children" in *Proceedings of the Sixth Minnesota State Conference of Charities and Corrections,* November 3–5, 1897, 72–76. Gillette's presentation was made within days of the admission of Royal Gray, the first child to receive care in the new hospital; "Free Treatment for Crippled and Deformed Children," *Northwestern Lancet* 18 (1898): 320–321; ibid., 19 (1899): 114–115, Boeckmann Library, St. Paul. These editorials were designed to inform physicians about the hospital, and they encouraged physicians to refer children for treatment.

14. *Minneapolis Journal,* August 6, 1898.

15. Editorial, "State Hospital for Crippled and Deformed Children" *The St. Paul Medical Journal* 1 (1899): 274–275, Boeckmann Library, St. Paul.

16. Frances Corning Boardman, "Report of Kindergarten Teacher," in *Second Annual Report of State Hospital for Crippled and Deformed Children, 1899,* (Minneapolis: Rice Bros. Printing Co., 1900), 3–16, GHP. Arthur Gillette's emphasis on education comes through in the inclusion of this information in the annual report.

17. University of Minnesota, Board of Regents, *Annual Reports of State Hospital for Crippled and Deformed Children,* 1898–1905, GHP; Board of Control, *Annual Reports of the Board of Control of St. Paul and Ramsey County,* 1904 and 1905, (St. Paul: The Pioneer Press Co.), Ramsey County Papers, MHS.

18. *House Journal,* State of Minnesota, H.F. No. 737, pp. 938–939, 1201, 1377, 1447, MSLL; *Senate Journal,* State of Minnesota, H.F. No. 737, pp. 914, 949, 951, 1030, 1064, 1073–1074, MSLL; *Laws of Minnesota for the Year of 1905,* Chapter 78, S.F. No. 114, p 95; idem, Chapter 203, S.F. No. 737, p. 257–258.

19. University of Minnesota, Board of Regents, *Annual Reports of State Hospital for Crippled and Deformed Children,* 1901–1906, GHP; Editorial, "Board of Control," *Northwestern Lancet* 21 (1901): 107. The author discusses the medical community's concerns regarding the appointment of a political board to manage fiscal matters of medical charities; Solon J. Buck, *The Autobiography and Letters of a Pioneer of Culture,* (Minneapolis, University of Minnesota Press, 1933), p. 242. Letter from Folwell to Mrs. Thomas R. Lounsbury, August 9, 1903, MHS. The author, president of the University of Minnesota, provided an example of faculty opinions regarding the Board of Control's fiscal management of state institutions: "The Regents nor any official cannot buy a sheet of paper, nor a ball of twine, but must apply to the Board of Control and satisfy that Board of the propriety of the expenditure. . . . If I were a member of the Board of Regents I would not serve another day"; Greenleaf Clark, "13th Annual Report of the Board of Regents of the University of Minnesota," *Minnesota Executive Documents,* 1903–04, Vol. IV, 398–399, MSLL. The Board of Regents submitted a formal request to be released from management of the Board of Control; "Some Setbacks," *The Charities Review,* Vol. IX, 1899–1900, (New York: The Charities Review) 57, MHS. The management of charitable organizations by state appointed boards, and specifically the Minnesota Board of Control, was discussed in a national forum.

20. University of Minnesota, Faculty Committee of the College of Medicine and Surgery Minutes, December 7, 1906, UMA. "Dean Wesbrook announced that Dr. Gillette had informed him on leaving that he would return before close of the Faculty, and that he would send a written notice to each member of the Faculty of the statement he had to make relating to the matter of locating the building for crippled and deformed children." The matter was referred to the Executive Committee with the power to act. Dr. Gillette's position was never recorded in the minutes of the group; Board of Regents Minutes, February 20, 1907, UMA; Board of Control, *Ninth Annual Report of State Hospital for Crippled and Deformed Children,* 1906, (St. Paul: The Pioneer Printing Co., 1905), GHP.

21. City of St. Paul, *Proceedings of the Common Council of the City of St. Paul, 1907,* A'y F No. 9395, Ramsey County, Board of Aldermen Papers, MSA. A resolution donating land owned by the State of Minnesota adjacent to City and County Hospital to build a hospital for crippled children.

22. "Industrial School for Crippled and Deformed Children," in *Biennial Report of the Minnesota State Board of Control to the Governor and the Legislature, 1906–07* and *1907–08,* Governor's Papers, MSA. Arthur Gillette's emphasis on education is clear: "Dr. A.J. Gillette, Surgeon of the institution, urges, with much force and reason, the establishment there of an Industrial School, . . . boy and girls may be taught such trades and occupations as will enable them to become self-supporting after they are finally discharged from the Hospital and School."

23. Ramsey County Clerk of Abstracts, 343170, condemnation statements for Phalen Park; idem, 323406, 610–616, Estate of Reuben Warner, March 9, 1906, Ramsey County Clerk of Abstracts, St. Paul; *The Commercial Club of St. Paul, 1893–1910,* (St. Paul: The Commercial Club, 1910), MHS; "Hospital is Needed for Little Unfortunates," *Pioneer Press,* August 19, 1906, MHS. Keeping the hospital in St. Paul became a matter of civic pride: "Men of this city are making an

earnest effort to do all in their power to interest men of wealth to contribute the sum needed to buy a suitable site and erect a building. Senator Dunn is actively engaged in the work of interesting men of St. Paul. He advocates and favors a site located near Phalen park. His plan is to secure the site through the beneficence of men of wealth in this city. . . . Many prominent men interested in charitable work have agreed to subscribe liberally. . . . This will require the hearty support of everyone, and since Hennepin county will have to be reckoned with, men who hope to secure the institution for St. Paul are diligently working to raise the necessary sum."

24. *Laws of Minnesota for the Year of 1907*, Chapter 81 – S. F. No. 526, 93–98. "An act to establish a state hospital for indigent, crippled and deformed children of the State of Minnesota, and to accept donations in aid thereof, and to provide for the management and control thereof, and authorizing the city of St. Paul to convey to the State of Minnesota certain lands as a site for such hospital"; Ramsey County Clerk of Abstracts, Deed of Conveyance, 349795 and 349796, Ramsey County, St. Paul. Documents the sale of remaining Warner property to the state.

25. *Laws of Minnesota for the Year of 1907*, Chapter 81; letters from L. A. Rosing, State Board of Control to J. C. Michael, city attorney, May 21, 1907 and August 19, 1907, MSA; letter from W. W. Dunn to J.C. Michael, city attorney, December 16, 1907, St. Paul City Attorney Correspondence, MSA.

26. *Laws of Minnesota for the Year of 1907*, Chapter 81.

27. State Board of Control, Minutes, May 27, 1907, Minnesota Board of Control Papers, Vol. A, MSA.

28. Arthur Ancker, M.D., "Report of Superintendent," *State Hospital for Crippled and Deformed Children*, 1908, (Minneapolis: Syndicate Printing Co.), GCSH.

29. Carl C. Chatterton, interview by Robert B. Winter, January, 1968, GSHC.

30. *Laws of Minnesota for the Year of 1909*, Chapter 130—S. F. No. 252. "An act to appropriate money for the purpose of constructing and equipping a Sanitarium and school building or buildings for the indigent, crippled and deformed children of the State of Minnesota, and for the care and education of such indigent, crippled persons as may be admitted to such Institution by the State Board of Control".

31. "Want State to Build. Should Erect Children's Home or Return Donated Site to Hospital," *Pioneer Press*, December 30, 1910, GHP. Members of the city council of St. Paul were irritated by the legislature's decision not to build the new hospital facility on land adjacent to City and County Hospital; Arthur Ancker, M.D., "Superintendent's Report," *Annual Report of The State Hospital for Indigent, Crippled and Deformed Children*, 1909, (Minneapolis: Syndicate Printing Company, 1910) 3, GCSH; *Laws of Minnesota for the Year 1911*, Chapter 195—S. F. No. 694, "An act to authorize and provide for the reconveyance to the City of St. Paul and the County of Ramsey, Minnesota, of certain lands conveyed to the State of Minnesota by said city and county under and pursuant to chapter 81 of the Laws of Minnesota for the year 1907, as a site for a state hospital for indigent, crippled and deformed children." Ultimately the city did regain control of the land adjacent to City and County Hospital that the City Council had given to the state as a site for the new children's hospital; Board of Control,

Annual Report of the Board of Control of St. Paul and Ramsey County for the Year Ending December 31, 1908.

32. Arthur Gillette, "Report of Surgeon-in-Chief," *Report and History of the Minnesota State Hospital and School for Indigent Crippled and Deformed Children to September 1, 1912* (St. Paul: The Pioneer Company) 7, GCSH.

33. Arthur Ancker, "Report of the City and County Physician," *Annual Report of the Board of Control of St. Paul and Ramsey County, 1914*, 48; Arthur Gillette, "Report of Surgeon-in-Chief," *Annual Report of the Minnesota State Hospital for Indigent Crippled and Deformed Children to August 1, 1914*, 6–8.

CHAPTER THREE: THE ORDER OF THINGS

1. Paul Clifford Larson, *Minnesota Architect: The Life and Work of Clarence H. Johnston* (Afton, MN: Afton Historical Society Press, 1996).

2. *Laws of Minnesota for the Year of 1909*, Chapter 130.

3. *Annual Report of The State Hospital for Indigent, Crippled and Deformed Children*, 1917; idem, 1918.

4. Ken Chowder, "How TB Survived Its Own Death To Confront Us Again," *Smithsonian* (1992): 180–194.

5. *Annual Reports of State Hospital for Crippled and Deformed Children*, 1897–1928, GHP.

6. Historical Research Collection, POA.

7. Board of Control, "Quarterly Conference of the Executive Officers of State Institutions with the State Board of Control at the State Hospital for Indigent, Crippled and Deformed Children, November 2, 1915," *Quarterly. Representing the Minnesota Education, Philanthropy and Penal Institutions* (Minneapolis: Syndicate Printing Co., 1915), MHS; idem, 1912–1928.

8. Donna K. Christianson, "Women in Minnesota—The McGregor Sisters," May 10, 1985, GCSH. Elizabeth and Margaret McGregor were the great aunts of Ms. Christianson.

9. Kathryn Gorman, "Portrait of a Children's Friend," *St. Paul Pioneer Press*, April 2, 1944, GHP.

10. Superintendent's Correspondence, 1911–1926, GHP; *Annual Report of the Minnesota State Hospital for Indigent Crippled and Deformed Children, 1916*, GCSH.

11. Christianson, "Women in Minnesota."

12. Jacob Zaun, "Sisters Kept Apart: Doctor Writes That State Hospital for Crippled Children Has a Cruel Rule," *St. Paul Dispatch*, July 24, 1920, MHS; letter from Elizabeth McGregor to Marie Diedenhofen, July 8, 1920, Superintendent's Correspondence.

13. Letters from H. M. Bracken, M.D., executive health officer, State Board of Health to Dr. Gillette, 1916–1918. Regarding epidemics and quarantines, Department of Health Papers, MSA; Editorial, "Influenza in Minnesota," *Minnesota Medicine* Vol. 4 (1920): 395–396; letter from John Marti, chief health inspector, City of St. Paul to State Hospital, January 9, 1925, small pox quarantine restrictions in 1925, GHP.

14. Jack Fincher, "America's Deadly Rendezvous with the 'Spanish Lady'," *Smithsonian* (1989): 130.

15. Carl C. Chatterton, interview by Robert B. Winter, January 1968, GSHC.

16. Letter from E. P. Lyon, dean of the medical school, to student interns, circa 1920, GHP. The letter outlines the

desired intern behavior while working at the university and other hospitals; "Rules and Regulations Governing Interns at the State Hospital for Indigent Crippled and Deformed Children," circa 1920s, GHP. This document details the responsibilities of interns during their assignment to hospital; Letters from Carl Chatterton to A. C. Strachauer, March 24, 1920. It seems the behavior of interns and students was a constant concern for Dr. Chatterton, who was beginning to assume more administrative responsibility at the hospital; E. P. Lyon, dean, the Medical School, February 14, 1922; Dr. A. Cameron, September 30, 1924, GHP.

17. *Annual Report of the Minnesota State Hospital for Indigent Crippled and Deformed Children*, 1909–1922.

CHAPTER FOUR: A HOME AWAY FROM HOME

1. From 1993 to 1997 the author received correspondence and conducted taped interviews of former and current patients, parents, and relatives. The information and stories in this chapter were developed from that information.

2. George Edmund Gilbertson, letter; George Edmund Gilbertson, *O Three Star* (Pasadena: unpublished, 1991). Glenn S. Erickson, letter; Glenn S. Erickson, *I Cried Three Times* (unpublished), POA.

3. Superintendent's Correspondence, 1911–1926; Carl C. Chatterton, interview by Robert B. Winter, January, 1968, GSHC.

4. Superintendent's Correspondence; Historical Research Collection, POA.

5. Gareth Hiebert, "1924 Christmas Love Still Burning," *St. Paul Pioneer Press*, December 29, 1974.

CHAPTER FIVE: THERE IS A SEASON

1. *Minneapolis Journal*, August 6, 1898.

2. Arthur J. Gillette, "The Presidential Address," *Northwestern Lancet* 17 (1987): 161–167; Editorial, "Honors for Minnesota," *St. Paul Medical Journal* (July 1900): 486; Edward Boeckmann, "The Ramsey County Medical Society—Its Past, Present, and Future," *St. Paul Medical Journal* (March, 1900): 147–170; Arthur J. Gillette, "The President's Address Before the Minnesota State Medical Association," *Minnesota Medicine* 1(10) (1918): 364–372; Arthur S. Hamilton, "An Historical Survey of the Minnesota Academy of Medicine," *The Journal-Lancet* XLV(10) (1925): 229–240.

3. University of Minnesota, Executive Committee, Board of Regents Minutes, September 13, 1915, UMA; idem, February 15, 1916.

4. J.A.A. Burnquist, "Arthur J. Gillette, M.D.," *Minnesota and its People*, Vol. IV, (The S. J. Clark Publishing Company, 1924).

5. Frederic G. Norton, letter to Dr. Larry Leider, September, 1971, GSHC; Frederic G. Norton, "On the Life of Doctor Arthur Gillette," September 6, 1971, GSHC.

6. C. Eugene Riggs, Robert Earl, and Wallace H. Cole, "Memorium to Dr. Gillette," *Minnesota Medicine* IV(6) (1921).

7. Superintendent's Correspondence, 1911–1926.

8. "Arthur J. Gillette," *Minneapolis Journal*, March 24, 1921.

9. Editorial, "Dr. Arthur Gillette," *The Journal-Lancet* April 1, 1921.

10. Emil Geist, "Arthur J. Gillette," *Minnesota Medicine*
IV(5) (1921): 326; R. O. Beard, "Arthur J. Gillette," *Minnesota Medicine* IV(5) (1921): 326; C. Eugene Riggs, Robert Earl, and Wallace H. Cole, "Memorium to Dr. Gillette," *Minnesota Medicine* IV(6) (1921).

11. *Laws of Minnesota for the Year 1925*, Chapter 61–S.F. No. 301; "Physicians Back Plan to Rename Hospital in Honor of Dr. Gillette," *St. Paul Pioneer Press*, 1923, GHP.

12. Carleton College, Annual Commencement Program, June 14, 1899, CCA; *The Spokane Directory*, 1899 through 1927; 1900 Federal Population Census, Eastern Washington Genealogical Society, P. O. Box 1826, Spokane, Washington, 99210.

13. Haskins, Jessie A., "A Page in a Man's Life," *The Carletonia* XVII (2) (1897): 4–6, CCA; Fones, (Ella and Jessie Haskins), *The Man With The Scar* (Boston: The Gorham Press, 1911); The Spokane Public Library, *Annual Reports 1908 and 1910*, Special Collections, Northwestern Room.

14. Letter from Maude Spear to F.H. Haggard, February 17, 1927, CCA.

15. Washington State Board of Health, Bureau of Vital Statistics, death certificate for Jessie Alice Haskins; Obituaries, *The Spokesman-Review* (Washington), February 8, 1927; Records, Hennessey-Smith Funeral Home and Crematorium, Inc., Spokane, Washington; Guide Map, Greenwood Memorial Terrace and Riverside Memorial Park, Spokane.

16. Michael John Dowling and Jennie Leonharda Bordewich Dowling Papers, MHS.

17. Michael J. Dowling, "A True Story of a Self Made Man. More Interesting and Fascinating Than Any Fiction," idem.

18. Superintendent's Correspondence; *Laws of Minnesota for the Year 1923*, Chapter 297.

19. Archives, GCSH; Grace Jones, interview by author, tape recording, Stillwater, MN, November 21, 1994; POA.

20. Board of Regents, Minutes, 1923, UMA.

21. Michael John Dowling and Jennie Leonharda Bordewich Dowling Papers, MHS.

22. Obituary, "Dr. Arthur B. Ancker," *Minnesota Medicine* VI (1923): 413; Mary Alice Czerwonka, "Roots of Ramsey's Health Care Trace Back to Ancker Hospital," *Ramsey County History* 22(1) (1987): 3–22; *The Journal-Lancet* 43 (1923): 281–2.

23. "Stephen Mahoney's Address," *The Minnesota Alumni Weekly* I (36) (1902): 19–21; "First Alumni Regent Dies," *The Minnesota Alumni Weekly* 32 (1932): 213.

CHAPTER SIX: THE TRADITION ENDURES

1. Letter from Downer Mullen to Elizabeth McGregor, May 11, 1921, Superintendent's Correspondence.

2. J. H. Moe and R. B. Winter, "Dr. Chatterton and Gillette Hospital," 1966, GCSH; "Cole-Chatterton Background," GCSH.

3. Carl C. Chatterton, interview by Robert B. Winter, January, 1968, CSH; Board of Control, *Annual Report of the Board of Control, City and County Hospital for the Year Ending 1938*.

4. Arthur J.Gillette and Carl C. Chatterton, "The Orthopedic Treatment of Deformities Resulting From Incurable Paralysis," *Minnesota Medicine* 1(1) (1918): 1–7.

5. *Minnesota State Hospital for Crippled and Deformed Children. Report for the Biennial Period Ending July 31, 1918.* GCSH.

6. Jean Conklin interview by author, tape recording, Bloomington, MN, January 17, 1994, POA.

7. Robert F. Premer, "A Gentleman Leads a Good Life," paper presented to the 25th meeting of The Wallace Cole Society, Pinehurst, North Carolina, October 15, 1993, GCSH. Dr. Premer was chief of orthopaedic surgery at the Minneapolis Veteran's Administration Hospital for more than thirty years and worked with Dr. Cole.

8. Board of Control, *Annual Report of the Board of Control, City and County Hospital for the Year Ending 1914*; Harry B. Hall, "Our Orthopaedic Personality: Wallace H. Cole, M.D," *The Bulletin of the American Academy of Orthopaedic Surgeons* 15 (17) (1967): 7–9, GCSH.

9. Wallace H. Cole, "The St. Paul Clinical Club, The St. Paul Medical Journal and Some Personal Reminiscences," paper presented to Min-Da-Man Orthopaedic Society, April 8, 1967.

10. Central States Orthopedic Club, Twin Cities-Rochester Meeting, October 11–13, 1915, GCSH.

11. Wallace H. Cole, "The St. Paul Clinical Club, op. cit.; Harry B. Hall, op. cit.; Robert F. Premer, op. cit.

12. Letters from Leonard F. Peltier to author, 1993. Minnesota Academy of Medicine Minutes, St. Joseph's Hospital Archives, St. Paul, MN; "Dr. Cole Back from War—6 Months in England," *St. Paul Pioneer Press*, September 5, 1942.

13. Leonard F. Peltier, "The Division of Orthopaedic Surgery in the A.E.F. a.k.a. The Goldthwait Unit," *Clinical Orthopaedics and Related Research* 200 (1985): 45–49. Wallace H. Cole, "The Story of Gillette Children's Hospital," 1972.

14. Wallace H. Cole, "The Use of the Thomas Bed Knee Splint for the Routine Treatment of Fracture of the Shaft of the Femur," *Minnesota Medicine* 1 (1920): 391–394.

15. Richard H. Jones, "A Fragment of Orthopaedic History," 1982, GCSH.

16. Jean Conklin interview.

17. Grace Jones interview.

18. Jean Conklin interview.

19. Interviews by author, 1993–1997, POA.; Grace Jones interview.

20. *Minnesota State Hospital for Crippled and Deformed Children, Biennial Reports,* 1916–1940, GCSH.

21. Letter from Elizabeth McGregor to C.E. Everett, November 23, 1923, Superintendent's Correspondence; Letter from Wallace H. Cole to Elizabeth McGregor, August 15, 1923, ibid.; Letter from Elizabeth McGregor to Mrs. Frank Walker, May 1, 1923, ibid.

22. State Board of Control, "Itemized Statement of Recommendations for Appropriations made by State Board of Control for the Department of Public Institutions," 1933, GCSH; State Board of Control, *Nineteenth Biennial Report of the State Board of Control,* State of Minnesota; *Seventh Biennial Report, Department of Public Institutions, Minnesota, 1938,* GCSH; State of Minnesota, Division of Public Institutions, *Biennial Reports,* 1940–1952, GCSH.

CHAPTER SEVEN: THE TIDAL WAVE

1. Maura Lerner, "Polio's Legacy," *Minneapolis Star Tribune,* June 19, 1996.

2. John R. Paul, *A History of Poliomyelitis* (New Haven and London: Yale University Press, 1971), 353.

3. Burton E. Aarness, letters home, 1922–23, POA.

4. Clara (Janzen) Trout, interview by Darla Stewart, tape recording, St. Paul, MN, October 23, 1993, POA.

5. Letter from Marjorie (Bassett) Simon to author, 1993.

6. Karen (Oberg) Valerius interview by Darla Stewart, tape recording, St. Paul, MN, September 30, 1993.

7. Paul, *History of Poliomyelitis.*

8. Robert W. Lovett, *The Treatment of Infantile Paralysis* (Philadelphia, P. Blakiston's Son and Co., 1916).

9. Victor Cohn, *Sister Kenny: The Woman Who Challenged the Doctors* (Minneapolis: The University of Minnesota Press, 1971); "Sister Kenny's Legacy," *Hennepin County History* 37(1) (1978): 3–14.

10. Bonita (Derby) Melzer interview by Darla Stewart, tape recording, St. Paul, MN, September 10, 1993, POA.

11. Elizabeth Cantwell interview by Darla Stewart, tape recording, St. Paul, MN, September 22, 1993, POA.

12. Beverly (Lyttle) Allstopp interview by Darla Stewart, tape recording, St. Paul, MN, February 2, 1994, POA.

13. Bonita Melzer interview.

14. Cohn, *Sister Kenny,* 4–5.

15. Letter from Wallace H. Cole to Elizabeth Kenny, 1940, GHP; W. H. Cole and M. E. Knapp, "The Kenny Treatment of Infantile Paralysis: A Preliminary Report," *Journal of the American Medical Association* 116 (1941): 2577–80.

16. Cohn, *Sister Kenny,* 6.

17. R. K. Ghormley, "Evaluation of the Kenny Treatment of Infantile Paralysis," *Journal of the American Medical Association* 125 (1944): 466–69; The report of Ghormley Committee, in part the result of the committee's visit to the University of Minnesota and Minneapolis General Hospital to view Sister Kenny's work, deeply offended her. Elizabeth Kenny Papers, MHS.

18. Letter from Elizabeth Kenny to Wallace Cole, December 4, 1946, Elizabeth Kenny Papers, MHS. Letter from Elizabeth Kenny to Wallace Cole, April 2, 1947, ibid.

19. Cohn, *Sister Kenny,* 8.

20. Historical Research Collection, POA.

21. Paul, *History of Poliomyelitis.*

22. Historical Research Collection, POA; Lois (Abramson) Johnson interview by Darla Stewart, tape recording, October 17, 1994, POA.

CHAPTER EIGHT: I REMEMBER

1. Historical Research Collection, POA.

2. Correspondence with author and interviews conducted by the author and Darla Stewart, tape recordings, St. Paul, Minnesota, 1993–1997, POA: Betty (Bowman) Atwood, Florence Bergvall, Karen (Bruber) Boche, Clair DeVries, Lowell O. Erdahl, Linda Fasching, Richard W. Foley, Carolyn (Ekelin) Freeberg, Alfred Gardner, Arliss (Klevenberg) Godejohn, Roger E. Gunderson, Richard L. Halversen, Larry E. Hayes, George W. Hofford, Richard F. Holt, Martha (Young) Ignaszewski, Lois (Abramson) Johnson, Beverly (Dixon) Krueger, Mary Ann (Carlin) Mulcrone, Mary (Bloom) Newman, Mary (Luce) Novak, Reba Radtke, Kathleen (Papenheim) Ramirez, Amanda Reimann, Elizabeth L. Reimann, Jeanette C. Steiner, John J.

Tobish, Karen (Oberg) Valerius, Nelvin L. Vos; George Hofford, *Recollections*, (San Jose: unpublished, July 1996).

    3. Historical Research Collection, POA.

    4. Op. cit.

CHAPTER NINE: MOUNDS OF MISERY

    1. Superintendent's Correspondence, GHP.

    2. Jean Conklin interview.

    3. Ibid., "Elizabeth McGregor, 74, Dies of Heart Ill," *St. Paul Dispatch*, April 1, 1950.

    4. Jean Conklin interview.

    5. Janet Hartman, tape recorded reminiscences, 1994, POA.

    6. Superintendent's Correspondence, GHP.

    7. Medical Staff Minutes, GCSH.

    8. Brendan Kennelly, guest speaker, "Presidential Address," at Scoliosis Research Society Annual Meeting, Dublin, Ireland, September 1993; Brendan Kennelly, "untitled poem," Spine 19 (14) (1994): 1549.

    9. Historical Research Collections, POA; Jean (O'Reilly) Wright, interviewed by Darla Stewart, tape recording, St. Paul, MN, August 27, 1993, POA.

    10. Historical Research Collection, POA.

    11. Historical Research Collection, POA; Robert B. Winter, tape recorded reminiscences, 1996, POA.

    12. Ibid.; Obituaries, "John H. Moe, M.D.," *Journal of Bone Joint Surgery* 70–A: (1988): 1577.

    13. Robert B. Winter, reminiscences.

    14. Historical Research Collection, POA; Robert B. Winter, reminiscences.

    15. Scoliosis Research Society, Membership Directories, (Park Ridge, IL:SRS); Robert B. Winter, reminiscences.

    16. Robert B. Winter, reminiscences.

    17. J. Martin Carlson, tape recorded reminiscences, April 1996, POA.

CHAPTER TEN: CARVING A NICHE

    1. *Laws of Minnesota for the Year 1959*, Chapter 262–H.F. No. 327.

    2. Medical Staff Minutes, December 16, 1961, GCSH.

    3. Ibid, February 2, 1963

    4. Ibid, July 20, 1963

    5. Jean Conklin interview, POA; James Hamilton and Associates, *"A Program of Development, Gillette State Hospital"* (Minneapolis: Hamilton Associates, 1966), GCSH.

    6. United States Government, Public Law 89–97 (Title XIX—Medicare); Hamilton and Associates, GCSH.

    7. Medical Staff Minutes, December 10, 1966.

    8. Letter from Morris Hursh to Senator William Kirscher, Senate Committee on Public Welfare, July 25, 1968, GCSH; Exhibit B, Report submitted by Dr. John Moe and Jean D. Conklin, to Welfare Sub-Committee, 1968, GCSH; letter from Jean Conklin to Senator Kirscher, 1968, results of survey; Robert Whereatt, "Hursh Backs Gillette Closing, Transfer of Orthopedic Program," *St. Paul Dispatch*, October 27, 1969; Transfer Urged for Gillette State Hospital, *Minneapolis Tribune*, October 28, 1969; "Gillette Staff Said to Favor Rebuilding," *St. Paul Pioneer Press*, October 28, 1969; *Laws of Minnesota for the Year of 1971*, Chapter 964–Subd. 15; ibid, Chapter 92–S.F. No. 291.

    9. Gillette Children's Hospital Papers, St. Paul; Clifford Retherford Papers, POA.

    10. *Laws of Minnesota for the Year of 1973*, Chapter 540–S.F. No. 56.; Gillette Children's Hospital Papers; Ozzie St. George, "Gillette Hospital Starts Big Move Monday, *St. Paul Pioneer Press*, April 10, 1977.

    11. Jean Conklin interview; *"Jean Conklin Day,"* Governor's Correspondence, MSA; Ozzie St. George, "Gillette Losing its Guiding Hand," *St. Paul Pioneer Press*, January 22, 1978.

    12. Gillette Children's Hospital Papers.

    13. Ibid.; Walter Parker, "Gillette Children's Hospital to Cut Staff by 20 Percent," *St. Paul Pioneer Press and Dispatch*, April 22, 1986; *Laws of Minnesota for the Year 1986*, Section 250.05; Walter Parker, "Minneapolis Children's to Manage Gillette Hospital," *St. Paul Pioneer Press* and *Dispatch*, December 22, 1986.

    14. Margaret Perryman, taped reminiscences, St. Paul, MN, April 1997.

    15. Gillette Children's Hospital Papers; *Laws of Minnesota for the Year 1988*, S. F. No. 2017, Section 250.05.

    16. Gillette Children's Hospital Papers.

    17. Maggie Tacheny, "Humanities Commission Ready to Move to East Side," *The East Side Review* (St. Paul), January 15, 1996.

CHAPTER ELEVEN: SIMPLY LISTENING

    1. Historical Research Collection, POA.

    2. Correspondence with author and interviews conducted by the author and Darla Stewart, tape recordings, St. Paul, Minnesota, 1993–1997, POA: Dina Blummer, Terry Blummer, Marian Bonkowske, Cheryl Brandes, James Brandes, Karen Goken, Terry Goken, Annette Lemke, Mary Kay O'Rourke, Molly O'Rourke, Kathy Orton, Steve Orton, Lynn Rodby, Scott Rodby.

    3. Don Boxmeyer, "A Nice Night For a Spin," *St. Paul Pioneer Press*, May 29, 1996.

CHAPTER TWELVE: APPLYING THE LESSONS

    1. Prologue, Rule of St. Benedict (multiple publishers over the centuries).

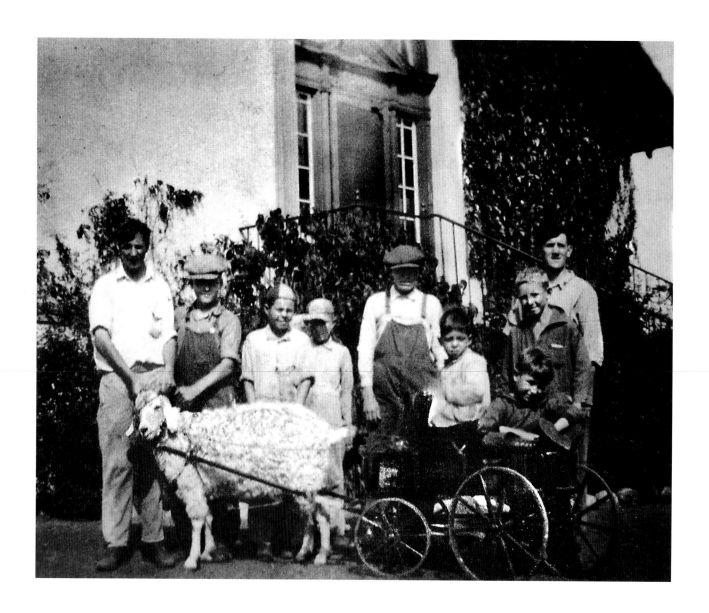

Appendix A

Chiefs Of Staff

Arthur J. Gillette (1897-21)
Carl C. Chatterton (1921-55)
Wallace H. Cole (1955-58)
John H. Moe (1958-73)
Wayne W. Thompson
(1973-1979)
Richard J. Aadalen
(1979-80)
James H. House (1981-82)
Robert B. Winter (1983-84)
Lowell D. Lutter (1985-86)
John E. Lonstein
(1987-1988)
Harry J. Robinson (1989-90)
Steven E. Koop (1991-92)
Linda E. Krach (1993-94)
Stephen B. Sundberg
(1995-96)
Steven E. Koop (1997-98)
Tom F. Novacheck
(1999-2000)

Medical Directors

Robert B. Winter
(1968-1980)
Keith D. Vanden Brink
(1980-86)
Robert B. Winter
(1986-1990)
James R. Gage
(1990-present)

Hospital Administrators

Arthur B. Ancker
(1907-1914)
Superintendent
Elizabeth McGregor
(1914-1949)
Superintendent

Jean Conklin
(1949-1977)
Administrator
Joseph Brown
(1977-1978)
Administrator
Norman Allan
(1978-1986)
Administrator
Margaret Perryman
(1986-present)
President/Chief
Executive Officer

Medical Staff

Richard J. Aadalen
Andrew Abramowitz
Frank Adair
Peter Agapitos
Gerald Ahern
David Ahrenholz
Hollis Ahrlin
Michael Ainslie
Behrooz Akbarnia
Max W. Alberts
H. J. Aldrich
Jeffrey Aldridge
Jeffrey Alexander
Hossein Aliabadi
C. S. Allen
Charles Alward
Michael Amaral
Arthur B. Ancker
Glen Anderson
Paul R. Anderson
Stanley Antolak
Nicholas I. Ardan, Jr.
H. C. Arey
Earl N. Armbrust

John Milton Armstrong
David Arnold
Mussarat Arshad
Narayan Athi
William G. Atmore
Mable F. Austin
Gary H. Baab
Frank S. Babb
Gilbert A. Bacon
G. W. Bagby
Walter L. Bailey
P. L. Baker
A. E. Baldwin
Charles R. Ball
Carol Ball
Evan Ballard
Bruce Bartie
Melissa Barton
W. C. Bason
Ronald Bateman
Eugene L. Bauer
A. Samuel Baumel
W. D. Beadie
Norman Beck
John Beer
Alfred F. Behrens
Arthur Beisang
C. A. Bell
John W. Benton
Luthard Bergh
M. Berkemann
F. Blanton Bessinger
Anthony Bianco
William H. Bickel
Claude W. Bierman
Paul Bigeleisen
H. E. Binger
David Binstaft
Roland C. Birkebak
Tobias Birnberg

R. G. Bjornson
Clyde E. Blackard
Jack Blaisdell
Peter Blasco
John W. Bloemendaal
Robert Blum
Karen Blumberg
Stephen Blythe
Joseph Bocklage
Lawrence R. Boies
David Borgstrom
Bernard Borkon
David S. Bradford
Albert G. Brandt
Elwyn R. Bray
William Brennom
J. B. Brimhall
Robert C. Brown
Walter M. Brown
Robert Bruce
Roy Bryan
Ronald Buck
Wilton H. Bunch
Victoria Buoen
Frank E. Burch
John Burkus
J. S. Burleigh
R. J. Burleson
Wesley H. Burnham
Michael F. Callaghan
Robert A. Callewart
Daniel R. Campbell
Terrance D. Capistrant
L. W. Carlander
W. A. Carley
W. W. Carroll
Alexander Cass
Reynaldo Castillo
Paul Cederberg
Carl C. Chatterton

167

M. H. Christensen
Lynn Christianson
James T. Christison
Roger Clausnitzer
J. Clayburgh
Woodward Colby
Wallace H. Cole
H. G. Collie
Alexander R. Colvin
Sarah Colwell
Thomas Comfort
George Constans
Paul Cook
David Cornfield
Aidan Cosgrove
Mark Coventry
K. W. Covey
Robin Crandall
Ray Critchfield
Kenneth Cross
Kent Crossley
James Crowe
Raul Cruz-Rodriquez
L. G. Culver
Bruce L. Cunningham
L. C. Dack
Mark T. Dahl
David A. Dassenko
E. B. Daugherty
Sandra Davenport
John G. Davidson
Elizabeth Davis
Eunice A. Davis
Richardo Delvillar
Francis Denis
Warren A. Dennis
Lizbeth Depadua
Ronald Dietzman
R. John Dittrich
Paul Donahue
Philip F. Donahue
John A. Dowdle
Thomas Dressel
Jack Drogt
Yadranko Ducic
Mary Beth Dunn
Ann C. Dunnigan

Arthur W. Dunning
Jay I. Durand
Everette J. Duthoy
L. A. Dwinnell
George Earl
Robert Earl
H. L. Eder
G. Edlung
Laura E. Edwards
James Egbert
C. T. Eginton
George Eichler
Vincent E. Eilers
Robert B. Elliott
Evan Ellison
Edward Emerson
Edward J. Engberg
Stephen P. England
Shoshana
    Englard-Falconer
Cesar Ercole
Donald L. Erickson
Andrew Erlanson
Henry Ernst
Julius O. Esho
Steven Eyer
David Falconer
Ralph Faville
D. A. Felder
David Ferenci
James C. Ferguson
John C. Feuling
Robert H. Fielden
Brian Fiedler
Dana Filipovich
Alfred Fish
Steven Fisher
Albert E. Flagstad
G. Flemming
Louis L. Flynn
William T. Flynn
John E. Foker
F. E. B. Foley
James D. Foley
Forrest Foreman
Mark Fox
Charles D. Freeman II

John F. Fulton
C. R. Gabbert
James R. Gage
Donald Gaines
Herbert Galloway
William F. Ganz
Gregory S. Garbin
V. Garcia
D. G. Gardner
Walter Gardner
John R. Gates
John Geiser
Emil Geist
Robert W. Geist
J. D. Geissinger
Steven Genheimer
Robert Giebink
Arthur J. Gillette
P. H. Gislason
Ronald J. Glasser
Paul Gleich
Jennifer W. Gobel
Meyer Z. Goldner
Ricardo Gonzales
Robert J. Gorlin
Mark E. Gormley
Robert J. Graham
Russell B. Graham
Lewis J. Gramer
R. D. Granquist
Richard Gray
Eric W. Green
Kathryn Green
Charles Lyman Greene
Allan Greenwood
Deborah Greenwood
Richard S. Gregory
J. F. Gross
Kent J. Gulden
J. L. Gulley
Robert J. Gumnit
Jerold Gurley
Ramone Gustillo
P. O. Gustafson
Jeffrey Haasbeek
Richard N. Hadley
George K. Hagaman

Erik Hakanson
Phillip Haley
A. R. Hall
Harry B. Hall
J. E. Halpin
David Hamlar
Ernest M. Hammes
Juliet R. Hanson
Rae Hanson
David Hardten
Paul R. Hartig
John Hartwig
Rise Hatten
Rolf Hauck
Julie Hauer
Fred Hayes
Albert C. Heath
John Heller
F. G. Hedenstrom
Melvin S. Henderson
W. H. Hengstler
Charles N. Hensel
E. T. Herrmann
G. J. Hiebert
Robert Hildebrandt
Joan Hilden
Thomas Hildreth
D. D. Hilger
Peter A. Hilger
J. J. Hinchey
Jane Hodgson
Alfred Hoff
C. W. Hogan
Jay Hollander
Robert W. Holmen
R. B. Holt
L. T. Hood
N. W. Hoover
James H. House
Alice Hulberg
Thomas Huseby
Vivian Husnik
Kano Ikeda
Allan Ingenito
Stephen M. Inglis
Gerald Ireland
Richard J. Ivance

John C. Ivins
F. J. Iwersen
A. E. Jackson
Joseph M. Janes
Steven Janousek
James E. Johanson
Byron Johnson
H. Paul Johnson
Harry A. Johnson
Lyle O. Johnson
Richard J. Johnson
Terry Johnson
Thomas J. Johnson
W. E. Johnson
Edward T. Jones
Grace Jones
Richard H. Jones
Deepak Kamat
Gordon Kamman
Nancy Kammer
William Kane
Edith Kang
Yale C. Kanter
C. I. Karleen
Clifford Kashtan
Elmer Kasperson
Sidney Kass
Harry I. Katz
S. W. Keck
Edward H. Kelly
P. J. Kelly
William A. Kennedy
Ansar U. Khan
Phillip Kibort
R. F. Kimbrough
Walter W. King
Rudolph A. Klassen
Henry N. Klein
Michael F. Koch
Rebecca Koerner
Daniel Kohen
Steven E. Koop
Gerald W. Koos
Leslie Kopietz
Richard Kowalsky
Linda E. Krach
J. D. Kramer

Robert L. Kriel
William J. Kube
Paul Kubic
M. G. Kunkel
D. M. Lafond
Sheldon M. Lagaard
Charles C. Lai
B. J. Lannin
V. G. La Rose
Louis Larsen
Carl L. Larson
Robert L. Larson
Andrew Lasky
Joseph Lee
R. M. Leick
Lloyd Leider
Arnold S. Leonard
William Lerche
Robert Leslie
N. Logan Leven
Richard Levinson
Carolyn Levitt
Royce C. Lewis
W. W. Lewis
E. Alexander L'Heureux
Philippe L'Heureux
A. G. Liedloff
L. Lima
Ronald L. Linscheid
Meryl Lipton
Jeffrey Lobas
George Logan
John E. Lonstein
Ernesto Lopez
Thomas A. Love
Charles Lukinac
John B. Lundseth
Lowell D. Lutter
Francis Lynch
Charles MacDonald
Archibald MacLaren
J. H. Madden
E. R. Maier
Bernard Maister
Barbara Malone
Charles Manlove
Richard Marnach

Steven Martin
Timothy Massey
John K. Matsuura
John R. Mawk
Robert Maxwell
Jack K. Mayfield
Donovan L. McCain
Sean McCance
F. E. McCaslin
Robert McClelland
N. C. McCloud
Randolph McConnie
James McCord
Paul McCormick
Thomas McDavitt
W. J. McDonald
Edward C. McElfresh
Michael McGonigal
N. A. McGreane
Carolyn J. McKay
C. Richard McKinley
Neil McLean
Felix McParland
Joseph Meade
J. P. Medelman
O. F. Melby
Mario Mendez
D. C. Meridith
G. L. Merkert
Robert L. Merrick
Michael A. Messenger
Michele Metrick
Christopher Meyer
E. A. Meyerding
Blaine Miller
W. C. Mitchell
Timothy Mjos
John H. Moe
Christopher Moertel
Paul Molinari
David Moore
James E. Moore
R. A. Morrill
Albert Mowlem
Robert A. Murray
Robert D. Mussey
Lance Mynderse

Mahmoud Nagib
Unni Narayanan
Teodoro Navarro
Joseph P. Neglia
David J. Nelson
George E. Nelson
J. Daniel Nelson
L. A. Nelson
Richard P. Nelson
James Nettleton
Roland F. Neumann
Karl Newman
E. H. Norris
Tom F. Novacheck
Malvin J. Nydahl
Orville E. Ockuly
Warren Ogden
James W. Ogilvie
Elias Olafsson
D. L. Olson
Dale V. Olson
Donald Olson
R. L. O'Neil
Betty Ong
E. H. O'Phelan
R. S. Osterholm
Frederick M. Owens
Julie Pagel
Jack Pascholl
Richard Patterson
Marshall E. Pedersen
L. G. Peltier
Michael Pergament
Joseph Perra
C. G. Perry
John Perry
Garry F. Peterson
Jonathan Phillips
Frank T. Pilney
Arnulf R. Pils
Wilbert Pino
Manuel Pinto
Charles A. Porretta
Edmund A. Post
James Prall
Robert Premer
Leland Prewitt, Jr.

Lumir C. Proshek
Sherrill Purves
Matthew Putnam
Deborah Quanbeck
Frank W. Quattlebaum
Mario Quinones
Olaf Raaen
Thomas J. Raih
Manuel Ramirez-Lassepa
Walter R. Ramsey
Cynthia Rask
Joseph M. Regan
Richard E. Reiley
Yuri Reinberg
Jose C. Reyes
R. Hampton Rich
Ernest T. F. Richards
Harold E. Richardson
Beverly Ricker
G. E. Ries
C. Eugene Riggs
Frank Rimell
Karen Ringsred
Harry Ritchie
Wallace P. Ritchie
Frank Ritter
Charles A. Roach
Stacy Roback
Myron Roberts
Harry J. Robinson
Charles Rogers
F. D. Rogers
Thomas F. Rolewicz
Frederick Rosendahl
Burton Rosenholtz
George N. Ruhberg
William Rupp
David Rustad
G. H. Ryan
Joseph Ryan
Michael Ryan
Edward L. Salovich
Shishikant Sane
John M. Scanlan
Dean Schamber
Marcus I. Schelander
Ivan Schloff

David Schmeling
Edward Schons
N. Joseph Schrandt
Warren Schubert
Sarah Schwarzenberg
Arnold G. Schwyzer
Sherwood B. Seitz
Michael Shannon
Ray M. Shannon
John L. Shellman
Phyllis Sher
Stewart W. Shimonek
James Sidman
Deanna Siliciano
Alan Sinaiko
Balbir Singh
D. G. Skagerberg
R. B. Skogerboe
Joseph I. Skow
Frank B. Smith
Michael Smith
Richard Smith
Robert Smith
Stephen Smith
Haldor Sneve
Bruce D. Snyder
Joseph J. Sockalosky
A. O. Sohanas
Robert Soiseth
Lynn D. Solem
John A. Soucheray
C. A. Spaulding
Edward D. Spear
Ivan M. Spear
Susan Spengler
Michael P. Sperl
Ronald H. Spiegel
Anton F. Spraitz
Paul Spray
Richard Stafford
John Stafne
Erik Stene
Joseph Stenzel
B. P. Stephens
Sheridan Stevens
Alexander Stewart
Peter J. Strand

Gordon Strate
Richard G. Strate
Gregg Strathy
Kevin Strathy
E. D. Strech
Marlin Strefling
E. D. Strick
Raymond Struck
Ronald Suiter
R. Sullivan
Jerald Sultz
Bruce Sundberg
Stephen B. Sundberg
Ian Swatez
Claude R. Swayze
Edward Szachowicz
Reginald Tall
Joseph Tambornino
Taro Tanaka
Marshall Taniguchi
Robert Telander
Soe M. Thein
Phudiphorn Thienprasit
Roby C. Thompson
Wayne W. Thompson
R. Thorton
Nancy Thorvilson
Christopher Tolan
Lyle A. Tongen
James S. Travis
Francis Trost
Daniel Tynan
R. M. Ulery
Jackson Upshaw
Mark Urban
Robert Vaaler
Fredrick Van Bergen
R. E. Van Demark
Ann Van Heest
Paul S. Van Puffelen
F. W. Van Slyke
Keith D. Vanden Brink
J. Howard Varney
Richard Vehe
A. E. Venables
Homer D. Venters
R. Vinjie

Norman L. Virnig
Roger Vitko
Dawn M. Voegeli
Victoria Volkova
William H. von der Weyer
Judith Wade
John Waldron
Albert Walnick
A. C. Walsh
W. H. Walton
Edmund L. Warren
Margaret Warwick
Richard Waterbury
John Wedge
John Weigelt
Darrell Weinman
George Weir
Joseph Wels
M. William Wheeler
James White
Daniel Whitlock
Paul Wicklund
George A. Williamson
Kent Wilson
O. Winter
Robert B. Winter
Sarah Winter
Michael Wipf
Peter Wirtz
C. F. Wohlrabe
James Wolpert
Kirkham Wood
Mark Yerby
M. A. Youel
Terri Young
Max R. Zarling
Joseph W. Zeleny
Samuel Ziegler
Judith Zier

This list of medical staff over
the last century was created
from a variety of hospital
documents. The author
apologizes for any omissions
and or inaccuracies.

Appendix B

APPLICATION BLANKS RECEIVED AT GILLETTE
STATE HOSPITAL 7-20-39.

Minnesota State Board of Control

#S352   Gillette State Hospital ——— Division of Services for Crippled Children

St. Paul, Minnesota

PHYSICIAN'S REPORT

Date _7-17_ 19_39_

Patient's Name _Hermanutz, Eugene, Irvin_   Address _Rockville, Min_
(Last) (First) (Second)

Date of Birth _12-23-32_   Male ☒ Female ☐   White ☒ Colored ☐ Indian ☐ Mexican ☐ Other ☐

Education   Grade School ①–2–3–4–5–6–7–8—   Other training

(Circle high-   High School 1–2–3–4—   Religion _Catholic_

est grade)   College 1–2–3–4—   Occupation _Student_

Father's name _Albin Hermanutz_   Nationality _German_   Place of Birth _Cold Spring, Minn_

Mother's maiden name _Elizabeth Waltz_   Nationality _"_   Place of Birth _Watkins, Minn_

BIRTH: Full term ☒ Premature ☐   Delivery: Normal ☐ Prolonged ☒ Instrument ☐ Other ☒ – _Podalic version_

Post-natal history: Convulsions ☐ Hemorrhage ☐ Cyanosis ☐ _difficult - large baby._

Development: First teeth _8_   Walked alone _1¼_   Talked _2 yrs_   Controlled bladder _3 yrs_   Bowels _3 yrs_
Age Age Age Age Age

Immunization and Vaccination: Diphtheria _0_   Material used
Age

Small Pox _0_   Other
Age

Previous Illnesses: (Check those which patient has had and give *age* at which illness occurred).

AGE	AGE	AGE	AGE
Chicken Pox	Influenza _6½ yrs_	Pneumonia	Small Pox
Chorea	Measles _6 mos ago_	Poliomyelitis	Tuberculosis
Diphtheria	Meningitis	Rheumatism	Typhoid Fever
Epilepsy	Mumps	Scarlet Fever	Whooping Cough

Cause (in parent's own words) _Birth Trauma_   Date disability began _Birth_

Nature of disability _Erb's palsy left_

Parts of body affected (specify R. and L.) _Left arm_

Previous medical care for disability(Give doctors' or hospitals' names and dates) _none_

Appliance worn at present: Yes ☐ No ☐ Type _none_

Present complaint _Unable to control left arm._

Tentative diagnosis _Erb's palsy (left)_

Treatment recommended: _Physiotherapy — Hospitalization_

(Specify hospitalization ☒ or out-patient department care ☐)

To your knowledge is this patient or his parents financially able to provide private orthopedic or plastic care? Yes ☐ No ☒

Signature of physician _Herman E. Koop_ M.D.

Address _Cold Spring, Minn_

An example of a referring physician's report, as completed by the author's grandfather, Dr. Herman E. Koop, Sr.

Appendix C

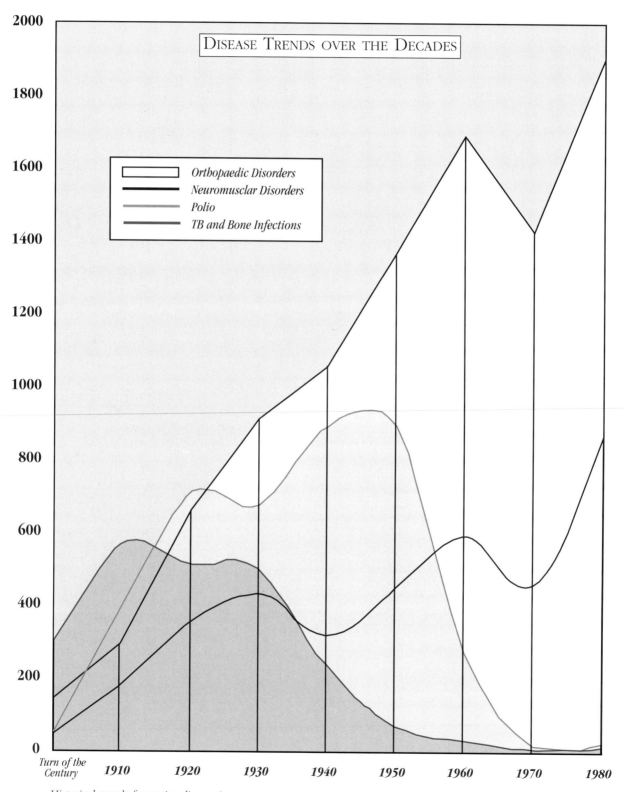

Historical trends for major diagnosis groups

Appendix D

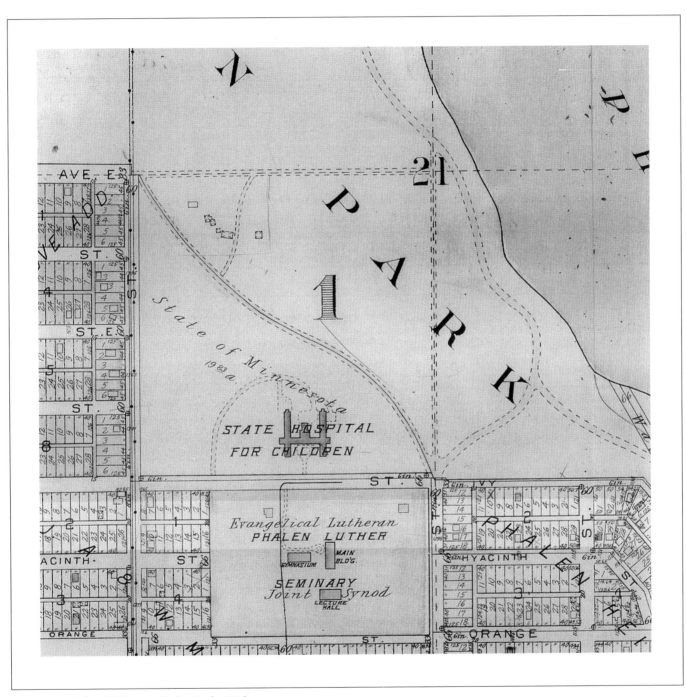

State Hospital for Children at Phalen Park, 1916

Index

Sources of Illustrations

CCA   Carleton College Archives, Northfield, Minnesota

GCH   Gillette Children's Hospital Historic Collection, St. Paul, Minnesota

MHS   Minnesota Historical Society, St. Paul, Minnesota

MHSG Minnesota Historical Society, Gillette Hospital Archives, St. Paul, Minnesota

POA   Pediatric Orthopaedic Associates, Historic Research Collection, Gillette Children's Hospital, St. Paul, Minnesota

RCMS Ramsey County Medical Society, Minneapolis, Minnesota

UMA   University of Minnesota Archives, Minneapolis, Minnesota

SPP

Cover: GCH
ii. Jean (Schilling) Legried photo; POA
iv. MHS
viii. GCH
2. CCA
3. *Carleton Ways and Byways and the Class of '99*, Northfield, Minnesota, 1899; CCA
4. GCH
5. CCA
8. RCMS
9t. C. P. Gibson photo; MHS
9b. UMA
11. Verna (Pratt) Host photos; POA, GCH
12. C. P. Gibson photo; MHS
13. GCH
16. *Men of Minnesota*, Minnesota Historical Co. publisher, 1902; MHS
17t. GCH
17b. RCMS
18t. GCH
18b. "State Care of Indigent Cripple and Deformed Children", Dr. Arthur Gillette, *St. Paul Medical Journal*, 1900; GCH
19. MHS
20. UMA
21. MHS
22. MHS
23. GCH
24. GCH
25. GCH
26. *Men of Minnesota*, 1902; MHS
27. "The Importance of Caring For, and How the State of Minnesota Cares for Its Indigent Children Suffering From Tuber-

culosis of the Bones and Joints", Dr. Arthur Gillette, *St. Paul Medical Journal*, January, 1909; GCH
29. GCH
32. MHS
33t. MHSG
33b. Gertrude (Honken) Albers photo; GCH
34. MHSG
35t. SPP
35b. GCH
36t. Robert Alva Shanor photo; POA
36b. A. F. Raymond photo; MHS
37. GCH
38. GCH
39t. Art Carlson photo; POA
39b. Art Carlson photo; POA
40. MHSG
41. GCH
42t. MHS
42b. MHSG
43. GCH
44. MHSG
45. GCH
46. Robert Alva Shanor photo; POA
48t. MHSG
48b. MHSG
49t. MHSG
49b. Art Carlson photo; POA
50t. MHSG
50b. MHSG
51. MHSG
52. GCH
53. MHSG
54t. MHSG
54b. GCH
55. MHSG
56. Rex Lambrecht photo; POA
57. Robert Alva Shanor photo; POA
58. GCH
59. SPP
60. Art Carlson photo; POA
61. Art Carlson photo; MHS
62. GCH
63. Jean (Schilling) Legried photo; POA
66. UMA
67. UMA
68. *Carleton Ways and Byways and the Class of '99*, CCA
70. Spokane Public Library, Northwest Room, Spokane, Washington
73. MHS
74. GCH
76. GCH
77. GCH
79. RCMS

80. GCH
82. Eleanor (Hable) Weiss photo; POA
83t. Joseph G. Baier photo; POA
83b. GCH
84. SPP
85t. GCH
85b. Marjorie (Bassett) Simon photo; POA
88. GCH
89t. Ernest Charley Johnson photo; POA
89b. Marjorie (Bassett) Simon photo; POA
90. Monica (Yanisch) Novotny photo; POA
91. MHS
93. Norma Fricke photo; POA
94. GCH
95. GCH
96. GCH
97. GCH
98. Lois (Abramson) Johnson photo; POA
99. Joseph G. Baier autograph book; POA
100. *1922 Biennial Report of State Hospital for Crippled and Deformed Children*; GCH
101. Glenn S. Erickson photo; POA
102t. GCH
102b. GCH
103. Charlotte (Allen) VanVleck; POA
104. GCH
105. Linda (Fasching) Ruhland photo; POA
106. GCH
107. MHSG
108. GCH
109. Linda (Fasching) Ruhland photo; POA
110. *1936 Biennial Report of Gillette State Hospital for Crippled Children*; GCH
111t. GCH
111b. MHSG
112. MHSG
113. SPP
116. GCH
117. GCH
118. GCH
119t. MHSG
119b. GCH
120. GCH
121t. GCH
121b. GCH
122. Rex Lambrecht photo; POA
123t. GCH
123b. GCH
124. GCH

125. GCH
126. GCH
127. SPP
130t. GCH
130b. GCH
131. GCH
132. GCH
133. GCH
134. GCH
135t. GCH
135b. GCH
136t. GCH
136b. GCH
137t. GCH
137b. GCH
138t. GCH
138b. GCH
139t. GCH
139b. GCH
142. GCH
143. GCH
144. Anna Bittner photo; GCH
145. Terri Poehls photo, St. Paul, Minnesota; GCH
146. GCH
147. GCH
148. Anna Bittner photo; GCH
149. GCH
150. GCH
151. GCH
153. Dorothy Brown photo, Hudson, Wisconsin
156. GCH
166. Henry Leslie Gustafson photo; POA
171. GCH
172. POA
173. Donald Empson, Empson Archives, Stillwater, Minnesota
Colophon page: GCH
Dust jacket flap: POA
Back cover: Henry Leslie Gustafson photo; POA

Contributors

Lorine (Anderson) Aandal
Burton Aarness
Dorothy Aarness
Sandra (Fischer) Adamski
Marjorie (Johnson) Airgood
Gertrude (Honken) Albers
Louise Albrecht
Beverly (Lyttle) Allstopp
Irene (Korpi) Almon
Lori J. Amerson
Marguerite (Bye) Andrews
Jeanne (Petschauer) Andrick
Betty (Bowman) Atwood
Gregory Averbeck
Marion Averbeck
Frank S. Baab, M.D.
Mary (Bazzachini) Baehr
Joseph G. Baier
Janet Marie Bailey
Gertrude (Vogt) Baran
Dora Barhaug
Loretta Beaver
Betty (Wemstrom) Bednarz
Ross Edwin Bengtson
Alva (Gow) Bergerson
Florence Bergvall
Janet Berndt
Kelly Berndt
William Bevins
Debra Lee Bieber
Joan (Savage) Billison
Patsy Jo Bishop
Pamela (Wallevand) Bjorklund
George R. Blank
Thomas M. Blomquist
Marcella (Sobczak) Blume
Maynard Blume
Dina Blummer
Katherine Blummer
Terry Blummer
Karen (Bruber) Boche
Irene (Gady) Boldt
Lenore Bolfing
Duane Q. Bondhus
Bradley Bonkowske

Marian Bonkowske
Roger Bonkowske
Anne (Hermanson) Boogroff
Cheryl Brandes
Ellen Brandes
James Brandes
Jerry Bredesen
Lucille C. Breen
Thomas A. Breen, M.D.
Ethel (Wold) Bristol
Dorothy Brown
Linda (Jasmer) Buhl
Esther (Carlson) Burkman
Lorene (Oslin) Burtts
Elizabeth Cantwell
Anne H. Carlsen
Art Carlson
Delaine Carlson
J. Martin Carlson
Jeffrey D. Carlson
Judith (Koenck) Carlson
Krista Christensen
Paul Erling Christensen
Lois Jean Christenson
Roger Christian
Alice (Wellcome) Clancy
Esther Clauson
Ada (Niemela) Collins
Jean Conklin
David K. Corrin
Vieno (Laulunen) Couville
Daniel Cowell
Eldon L. Coyle
Andrea (Rakowski) Crosby
Julia Cunningham
Carlee J. Dahl
Maureen DalCanton
Michael Lee DalCanton
Floyd L. Dean
Eugene DeBolt
Jessica Kay Dennis
Kay Dennis
Clair John DeVries
Charles Dillerud
Elder Dillerud
Constance (Cunningham)
   Dillon
Edith Donley
Beatrice Dorawa
Marvin Doucette
Emmaline (Polzin) Dunkley
Thomas G. Dunn

Marion L. Edgar
Charles T. Eginton, M.D.
Blanche (Williamson) Elf
Agnes Elkjer
Lowell O. Erdahl
Bonnie (Good) Erickson
Glenn S. Erickson
Darwin L. Ferrier
Sharon (Peterson) Fjestad
Richard W. Foley
Eugene L. Ford
Glenn W. Ford
Gilford Foslien
Adeline Fossen
Kimberly D. Frank
Donna Fredine
Carolyn Ann (Ekelin) Freeberg
Lorrie Lee Freund
Lia Frey-Rabine
Norma J. Fricke
Alfred Gardner
Marlene C. Gardner
James H. Garoutte
Opal Gartzke
Ella M. Gaulke
Lucille Geisinger
G. Edmund Gilbertson
Arliss (Klevenberg) Godejon
Karen S. Goken
Maxwell Goken
Terry Goken
Marie (Bassett) Gosewisch
Robert J. Gosselin
Eunice (Halvorson) Graham
Michael Graves
Leander C. Gresser
Bertie Lou (Behnen) Gruber
Beulah Guethlein
Roger E. Gunderson
Henry Leslie Gustafson
Roland R. Hagel
Gloria (Bishop) Haley
Amy (Syverson) Hallberg
Richard L. Halverson
James W. Hamilton
Peter E. Hansen
Margaret (Tauer) Hard
Nicholas Harens
Virginia Harens
Janet Hartman
Monica (Schmitt) Hartman
Brian Haugrud

Larry E. Hayes
Lois (Grupe) Heckman
Elsa Hedberg
Jeanette Heins
Agnes (Schermann)
   Henderson
Vernon A. Henk
Eugene Hermanutz
Evelyn (Cousins) Hermoe
Jennifer Hinds
Florence Hinsch
Fred Hinsch
Thomas Hinsch
Beauford Hintze
Joyce (Besser) Hippen
Clyde Annen Hirschey
Vera Hirschey
George W. Hofford
Margaret Holland
Lorna M. Holm
Richard F. Holt
Verna (Pratt) Host
James P. Howard
Hazel Louise Howe
Ed Huebsch
Helen Huebsch
Kathleen (Anderson)
   Husmann
Martha (Young) Ignaszewski
Violet (Carlson) Jackson
Carmen (Pilegaard) Jagt
Anne (Bozich) Jagunich
Mary E. (Beulke) Jahnke
David Russell Johnson
Earl V. Johnson
Ernest Charly Johnson
Jeanne M. Johnson
Lois (Abramson) Johnson
Lyle O. Johnson, M.D.
Rosemary (Ackermann)
   Johnson
Sharon (Osborn) Johnson
Patricia (Keller) Johnston
Dorothy (Lucking) Jones
Grace Jones, D.D.S.
Marion (Harrington) Jones
Bonnie Jostock
Anthony Julik
Delores Kaese
Robert E. Kick
Robert A. Kierlin
Ralph W. Kilker

Lawrence Klennert
Jay B. Knaak
Evelyn B. Knudson
Karol Kolb
Carla (Veenhof) Korthals
Leona Kroska
Beverly (Dixon) Krueger
Jeanette R. Kruger
Karen (Thornton) Krugerud
Norman Kuehne
Lorraine Kuperus
Jeffrey Kustritz
Judy A. Laatsch
Lorna (Kuehne) Lambrecht
Rex Lambrecht
Frances (Peck) Lammers
Diane (Oaks) Lande
Randy C. Larson
Mary (Bentler) Leader
Jean (Schilling) Legried
Steven L. Lehmann
Annette Lemke
Dennis Lemke
Lee Lemke
Karen (Dobson) Lewis
Richard P. Lilla
Mary Lindgren
Ruby (Koecher) Lodien
Melvin A. Loesch
Susan (Perleberg) Loscheider
Edward Kempton Lucking
John J. Ludden
Margaret M. Ludden
Duane N. Lundgren
William H. Lyttle
Barbara (Dietz) Macho
Marlene Mann
Bernice (Rudnitski) Marshik
Leila (Ely) Maxey
Kathleen McDougall
Renaye (Post) McDougall
Geraldine (Dougherty)
    McGhee
Alice (Peters) Meland
Bonita (Derby) Melzer
Julie Menken
Lorna Menken
Robert D. Meyer
Doris (Williams) Meyers
John H. Midtaune
Patricia (Anderson) Minaker
Carolyn Mischler
Gerald M. Modjeski
Rose (Borrell) Monahan
Jean (Perry) Mouchly
Dale R. Muehlbaum

Paul A. Mueller
Rick Muenich
Mary Ann (Carlin) Mulcrone
Richard S. Munson
Berneil C. Nelson
Elmer Henry Nelson
Gerald D. Nelson
Harold L. Nelson
Kelly (Krautkremer) Nelson
Norman H. Nelson
Michelle (Madsen) Ness
Linda Neste
Mary (Bloom) Newman
Audre (Styba) Noeske
Barbara (Kachinske) Norell
James Cornelius Norland
John Norland
Mary (Luce) Novak
Monica (Yanisch) Novotny
Susan R. Offerdahl
MerriKay Oleen-Burkey
Allan T. Olich
Gene Lester Olson
Merle Leroy Olson
Richard H. Olson
Donald L. Oman
Mary Kay O'Rourke
Molly O'Rourke
Steve Orton
Kathy Orton
Marcia (Rudie) Osberg
Mark Paakkonen
Patricia (Anderson) Paciotti
Beverly Y. Pederson
Ruth (Hunt) Perovsek
Carl Perpich
Deanna (Johnson) Perrine
Margaret E. Perryman
Adeline (Nyquist) Peterson
Carole Peterson
Eleanor (Bengtson) Peterson
Lucinda Peterson
Robert S. Peterson
Elsie (Laine) Piirainen
Nancy Pilegaard
Bernard Pirjevec
Ruth (Langan) Pitney
Pamela Ritchie Plummer
John M. Popp
Marilyn J. Pozel
Dwayne A. Puffer
Anthony T. Radaich
Mary Ellen (Mullaney)
    Radman
Nancy Lee Radtke
Reba Radtke

Kathleen (Papenheim)
    Ramirez
Sylvia S. Reasor
Bernard S. Reding
Janet (Quam) Reding
Monica Reilly
Amanda Reimann
Elizabeth L. Reimann
Michael Arthur Reimann
Mary Ann (Cortright)
    Reimersma
Rebecca (Loechler) Reitmann
Alice Retherford
Clifford Retherford
Everett Riedberger
Lynn Rodby
Robert Rodby
Steven Rodby
Scott Rodby
Eva (Hoehn) Rollins
Lois (Huebsch) Root
Melvie (Hippe) Ross
William Rossow
Daniel Rowe
Lillian (Zanoth) Rozeske
Linda (Fasching) Ruhland
Ronald E. Saatela
Judith (Olson) Schlingman
Charles B. Schmitz
Patricia (Ziska) Schmitz-Kulzer
Patricia (Sorgatz)
    Scholljegerdes
Roseann (Krall) Schomber
Rudell (Larson) Schroeder
Barbara Schueler
Joshua C. Schueler
Janice (Weinand) Schuster
Eleanor (Guethlein) Schwalbe
Terry (Kopp) Schwartz
Jane Sears
Eugene Selsvold
Joseph Shanor
Robert Alva Shanor
David Shaw
Allan Shelstad
Kirsten Shelstad
Henry Shogren
Marjorie (Bassett) Simon
Richard M. Skarman
Mildred Skoglund
Roger Sonied Skoglund
L. Paul Skogrand
Rodger N. Smalley
Bude Smilanich
Dale L. Smith
Audrey (Gruber) Snell

Elliott T. Sovell
Violet Spinler
Niki Lyn Squier
Kathleen Stanek
Tamera Stanek
Mildred (Hansen) Stangeland
Lois (Lindblom) Steffen
Jeanette C. Steiner
Joel Stenhaug
Doris Stewart
Grace Swenson
John P. Taney
June (Kuperus) Templer
John J. Tobish
James L. Tolan
Dorothy (Werner) Tompkins
Dorene (Dallmann) Trahan
June (Terhark) Tretbar
Clara (Janzen) Trout
Delores (Lanoux) Tschida
Barbara Ellen Tuttle
Karen (Oberg) Valerius
Charlotte (Allen) Van Vleck
Margaret (Damsgard) Veile
Bozana (Djuth) Verkovich
Irene (Hauge) Viken
Frank Vogt
Nelvin L. Vos
Chester A. (Weberg) Walker
Cleone F. (Rogers) Watkins
Willis (Rushenberg) Watson
Harold Weaver
Eleanor (Hable) Weiss
Robert C. Wig
Evelyn (Witter) Wilcox
Virginia (Zech) Williams
Elizabeth (Gawreluk) Wilson
Robert B. Winter, M.D.
Diane (Wittner) Wippler
Peter D. Wojcik
Geraldine (Fincel) Worth
Jean (O'Reilly) Wright
Charles Youngberg
Nina M. Youngberg
Carol Zielinski
Kathleen Rae Zondervan

The author apologizes for any
omissions and or inaccuracies.

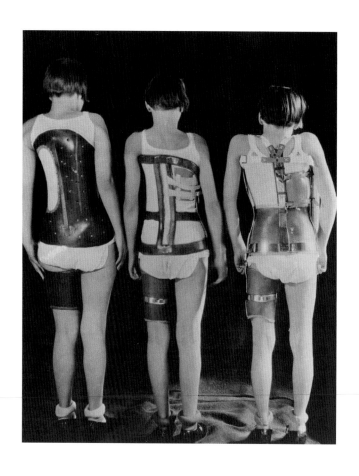

Designed by
Barbara J. Arney
Stillwater, MN

Typefaces are
Garamond and ExPonto